Precision Sleep Medicine

Editor

SUSHEEL P. PATIL

SLEEP MEDICINE CLINICS

www.sleep.theclinics.com

Consulting Editor
TEOFILO LEE-CHIONG Jr

September 2019 • Volume 14 • Number 3

ELSEVIER

1600 John F. Kennedy Boulevard • Suite 1800 • Philadelphia, Pennsylvania, 19103-2899

http://www.theclinics.com

SLEEP MEDICINE CLINICS Volume 14, Number 3
September 2019, ISSN 1556-407X, ISBN-13: 978-0-323-68216-9

Editor: Colleen Dietzler
Developmental Editor: Donald Mumford

Sleep Medicine Clinics (ISSN 1556-407X) is published quarterly by Elsevier Inc., 360 Park Avenue South, New York, NY 10010-1710. Months of issue are March, June, September and December. Business and Editorial Offices: 1600 John F. Kennedy Blvd., Ste. 1800, Philadelphia, PA 19103-2899. Customer Service Office: 3251 Riverport Lane, Maryland Heights, MO 63043. Periodicals postage paid at New York, NY and additional mailing offices. Subscription prices are $212.00 per year (US individuals), $100.00 (US students), $486.00 (US institutions), $264.00 (Canadian individuals), $252.00 (international individuals), $135.00 (Canadian and international students), $551.00 (Canadian institutions) and $551.00 (International institutions). Foreign air speed delivery is included in all *Clinics* subscription prices. All prices are subject to change without notice. **POSTMASTER:** Send change of address to *Sleep Medicine Clinics*, Elsevier Health Sciences Division, Subscription Customer Service, 3251 Riverport Lane, Maryland Heights, MO 63043. Customer Service: **Tel: 1-800-654-2452 (U.S. and Canada); 314-447-8871 (outside U.S. and Canada). Fax: 314-447-8029. E-mail: journalscustomerservice-usa@elsevier.com (for print support); journalsonlinesupport-usa@elsevier.com (for online support).**

Reprints. For copies of 100 or more of articles in this publication, please contact the Commercial Reprints Department, Elsevier Inc., 360 Park Avenue South, New York, NY 10010-1710. Tel.: 212-633-3874; Fax: 212-633-3820; E-mail: reprints@elsevier.com

Sleep Medicine Clinics is covered in *MEDLINE/PubMed (Index Medicus).*

SLEEP MEDICINE CLINICS

FORTHCOMING ISSUES

December 2019
Sleep and Transportation
Walter McNicholas, *Editor*

March 2020
Sleep and Performance
Rachel R. Markwald and Anne Germain, *Editors*

June 2020
Telehealth in Sleep Medicine
Jean Louis Pépin and Dennis Hwang, *Editors*

RECENT ISSUES

June 2019
Cognitive Behavioral Therapies for Insomnia
Jason C. Ong, *Editor*

March 2019
Prevention, Screening, and Treatments for Obstructive Sleep Apnea: Beyond Positive Airway Pressure (PAP)
Song Tar Toh, *Editor*

December 2018
Dental Sleep Medicine
Jamison R. Spencer, *Editor*

SERIES OF RELATED INTEREST

Clinics in Chest Medicine
Available at: https://www.chestmed.theclinics.com/

THE CLINICS ARE AVAILABLE ONLINE!
Access your subscription at:
www.theclinics.com

Contributors

CONSULTING EDITOR

TEOFILO LEE-CHIONG Jr, MD
Professor of Medicine, National Jewish Health,
University of Colorado Denver, Denver,
Colorado, USA; Chief Medical Liaison, Philips
Respironics, Pennsylvania, USA

EDITOR

SUSHEEL P. PATIL, MD, PhD
Clinical Director, Johns Hopkins Pulmonary
Sleep Medicine Program
Assistant Professor of Medicine
Johns Hopkins University School of Medicine
Division of Pulmonary and Critical
Care Medicine
Baltimore, Maryland, USA

AUTHORS

ISABELLE ARNULF, MD, PhD
National Reference Center for Rare
Hypersomnias, Pitie-Salpetriere University
Hospital, APHP, and Sorbonne University,
Paris, France

THOMAS J. BALKIN, PhD
Behavioral Biology Branch, Walter Reed Army
Institute of Research, Silver Spring, Maryland,
USA

ELAINE BOLAND, PhD
Department of Psychiatry, Perelman School
of Medicine of the University of
Pennsylvania, Michael J. Crescenz VA
Medical Center, Philadelphia, Pennsylvania,
USA

PATRICIA CARTER, PhD, RN, CNS
Associate Professor and Director, Leadership
in Diverse Settings Program, School of
Nursing, University of Texas at Austin, Austin,
Texas, USA

PAULINE DODET, MD
National Reference Center for Rare
Hypersomnias, Pitie-Salpetriere University
Hospital, APHP, and Sorbonne University,
Paris, France

JOEL ERICKSON, MD
Sleep Medicine Fellow, Department of
Neurology, University of North Carolina,
Chapel Hill, University of North Carolina School
of Medicine, Chapel Hill, North Carolina, USA

PHILIP R. GEHRMAN, PhD
Department of Psychiatry, Perelman
School of Medicine of the University of
Pennsylvania, Michael J. Crescenz VA
Medical Center, Philadelphia, Pennsylvania,
USA

JENNIFER GOLDSCHMIED, PhD
Department of Psychiatry, Perelman
School of Medicine of the University of
Pennsylvania, Philadelphia, Pennsylvania,
USA

BIRGIT HÖUGL, MD
Department of Neurology, Medical University
of Innsbruck, Innsbruck, Austria

STEVEN HURSH, PhD
Institutes for Behavior Resources, Inc,
Baltimore, Maryland, USA

ANNEMARIE IDA LUIK, PhD
Assistant Professor, Department of
Epidemiology, Erasmus MC University Medical
Center, Rotterdam, the Netherlands

ALEX IRANZO, MD
Neurology Service, Multidisciplinary Sleep
Unit, Hospital Clinic de Barcelona, Institut
D'Investigacions Biomèdiques August Pi i
Sunyer, Centro de Investigacion Biomedica en
Red de Enfermedades Neurodegenerativas,
Barcelona, Spain

MATTHEW S. KAYSER, MD, PhD
Department of Psychiatry, Perelman School of
Medicine of the University of Pennsylvania,
Philadelphia, Pennsylvania, USA

ANDREW D. KRYSTAL, MD, MS
Ray and Dagmar Dolby Distinguished
Professor, Director, Clinical and Translational
Sleep Research Program Director, Dolby
Family Center for Mood Disorders Director,
Interventional Psychiatry Program, Vice-Chair,
Research, Department of Psychiatry,
University of California San Francisco, San
Francisco, California, USA; Emeritus
Professor, Psychiatry and Behavioral
Sciences, Duke University School of Medicine,
Durham, North Carolina, USA

JAAP LANCEE, PhD
Assistant Professor, Department of Clinical
Psychology, University of Amsterdam, PsyQ
Amsterdam, Amsterdam, the Netherlands

SMARANDA LEU-SEMENESCU, MD
National Reference Center for Rare
Hypersomnias, Pitie-Salpetriere University
Hospital, APHP, and Sorbonne University,
Paris, France

MATTHEW LIGHT, MD
Fellow, Division of Pulmonary, Critical
Care and Sleep Medicine, University of
California San Diego, La Jolla, California,
USA

ATUL MALHOTRA, MD
Professor, Division of Pulmonary, Critical
Care and Sleep Medicine, University of
California San Diego, La Jolla, California, USA

ROBERT L. OWENS, MD
Associate Professor, Division of Pulmonary,
Critical Care and Sleep Medicine, University of
California San Diego, La Jolla, California, USA

ALLAN I. PACK, MBChB, PhD
Translational Research Laboratories, John
Miclot Professor of Medicine, Director, Center
for Sleep and Circadian Neurobiology,
University of Pennsylvania Perelman School of
Medicine, Philadelphia, Pennsylvania, USA

LUIS E. PICHARD, MHS, PhD
Division of Pulmonary and Critical Care
Medicine, Department of Medicine, The Johns
Hopkins University School of Medicine,
Baltimore, Maryland, USA

ARIC A. PRATHER, PhD
Associate Professor, Director, Behavioral
Sleep Medicine Program, Department
of Psychiatry, University of California
San Francisco, San Francisco, California, USA

KATHY RICHARDS, PhD, RN, FAAN, FAASM
Research Professor, School of Nursing,
University of Texas at Austin, Austin, Texas,
USA

JOAN SANTAMARIA, MD
Neurology Service, Multidisciplinary Sleep
Unit, Hospital Clinic de Barcelona, Institut
D'Investigacions Biomèdiques August Pi i
Sunyer, Centro de Investigacion Biomedica en
Red de Enfermedades Neurodegenerativas,
Barcelona, Spain

CHRISTOPHER N. SCHMICKL, MD, PhD
Fellow, Division of Pulmonary, Critical
Care and Sleep Medicine, University of
California San Diego, La Jolla, California, USA

LINDSAY SCHWARTZ, PhD
Institutes for Behavior Resources, Inc,
Baltimore, Maryland, USA

GUIDO SIMONELLI, MD
Behavioral Biology Branch, Walter Reed Army
Institute of Research, Silver Spring, Maryland,
USA

AMBRA STEFANI, MD
Department of Neurology, Medical University of Innsbruck, Innsbruck, Austria

VANI VALLABHANENI, MD
Board Certified in Sleep Medicine, Board Certified in Internal Medicine, Clinical Assistant Professor, Texas A&M University, College Station, Texas, USA; Medical Director, Sleep 360 Sleep Diagnostic Center, Austin, Texas, USA

TANJA VAN DER ZWEERDE, MSc
PhD-candidate, Department of Clinical Psychology, EMGO Institute for Health and Care Research, VU University, Amsterdam, the Netherlands

ANNEMIEKE VAN STRATEN, PhD
Professor, Department of Clinical Psychology, EMGO Institute for Health and Care Research, VU University, Amsterdam, the Netherlands

BRADLEY V. VAUGHN, MD
Professor, Department of Neurology, University of North Carolina, Chapel Hill, University of North Carolina School of Medicine, Chapel Hill, North Carolina, USA

LICHUAN YE, PhD, RN
Associate Professor, School of Nursing, Bouve College of Health Sciences, Northeastern University, Boston, Massachusetts, USA

Contents

Preface: Precision Medicine in the Field of Sleep Medicine: Early Days   xiii

Susheel P. Patil

Precision Medicine for Insomnia   291

Elaine Boland, Jennifer Goldschmied, Matthew S. Kayser, and Philip R. Gehrman

Insomnia affects up to 15% of the US population. There are effective pharmacologic and behavioral treatments for insomnia; however, there is often no one-size-fits-all intervention. This article discusses the leading behavioral treatment of insomnia, cognitive behavioral therapy for insomnia, and its ability to be tailored to an individual's specific symptoms. It then discusses pharmacologic options for treating insomnia, and offers some guidance on medication selection to enhance personalized care. In addition, it discusses how the current evidence base can help providers make choices between pharmacologic and behavioral treatments.

Internet-Delivered Cognitive Behavioral Therapy for Insomnia: Tailoring Cognitive Behavioral Therapy for Insomnia for Patients with Chronic Insomnia   301

Tanja van der Zweerde, Jaap Lancee, Annemarie Ida Luik, and Annemieke van Straten

Chronic insomnia is preferably treated with cognitive behavioral therapy for insomnia (CBTI), but many insomnia sufferers receive medication instead, likely because of high costs, lack of knowledge about optimal insomnia treatment among physicians, and lack of CBTI-trained professionals in mental health care. A possible solution is to offer CBTI through the Internet: I-CBTI. I-CBTI is generally acceptable to patients and greatly improves insomnia symptoms. We review the state of knowledge around I-CBTI and its effects. CBTI's effectiveness is influenced by treatment characteristics and patient-specific factors. We review potential factors that help identify which patients may benefit from I-CBTI.

Sleep Pharmacogenetics: The Promise of Precision Medicine   317

Andrew D. Krystal and Aric A. Prather

Pharmacogenetics is the branch of personalized medicine concerned with the variability in drug response occurring because of heredity. Advances in genetics research, and decreasing costs of gene sequencing, are promoting tremendous growth in pharmacogenetics in all areas of medicine, including sleep medicine. This article reviews the body of research indicating that there are genetic variations that affect the therapeutic actions and adverse effects of agents used for the treatment of sleep disorders to show the potential of pharmacogenetics to improve the clinical practice of sleep medicine.

Precision Medicine for Idiopathic Hypersomnia   333

Isabelle Arnulf, Smaranda Leu-Semenescu, and Pauline Dodet

Idiopathic hypersomnia (IH) is characterized by excessive daytime sleepiness despite normal or prolonged sleep. IH is distinguished from narcolepsy by the female predominance, severe morning inertia, continuous drowsiness (rather than sleep attacks), unrefreshing naps, absence of cataplexy, sleep onset in REM periods, and hypocretin deficiency. In IH, the multiple sleep latency test demonstrates low sensitivity, specificity, and reproducibility, compared with prolonged sleep monitoring. In some IH cases, an endogenous hypnotic peptide stimulating GABA receptors during wakefulness is suspected, which are improved by anti-GABA drugs. The benefits of modafinil, sodium oxybate, mazindol, and pitolisant were found in mostly retrospective studies.

Precision Medicine in Rapid Eye Movement Sleep Behavior Disorder   351

Birgit Högl, Joan Santamaria, Alex Iranzo, and Ambra Stefani

In recent years, the diagnostic approach to rapid eye movement (REM) sleep behavior disorder (RBD) has become more objective and accurate. This was achieved mainly by introduction of methods to exactly quantify electromyographic (EMG) activity in various muscles during REM sleep. The most established muscle combination for RBD diagnosis is the mentalis and upper extremity EMG. Computer-assisted systems for this analysis have been described, and an increasing number of studies looked into analysis of video events. Recently, prodromal phases of isolated RBD have been recognized.

Non-REM Parasomnia: The Promise of Precision Medicine   363

Joel Erickson and Bradley V. Vaughn

Our understanding of non-REM parasomnias is just beginning to unfold the potential biomarkers and underlying pathophysiologic processes that lead to these events. Biomarkers need further investigation and will help us to understand better ways to develop risk models and possible mechanisms. Similarly, as we develop more accurate pathophysiologic-based diagnostic testing for non-REM parasomnias, we will begin the evolution toward a physiologic-based classification scheme that aids the application of precision medicine. This article explores currently known characteristics and exploratory features that may aid in this transition to better understanding our individual patients with non-REM parasomnias and tailoring their treatments.

Sleep and Memory: The Promise of Precision Medicine   371

Patricia Carter, Lichuan Ye, Kathy Richards, and Vani Vallabhaneni

Given the complex and bidirectional nature of sleep and mild cognitive impairment/ Alzheimer's disease and related dementias, a precision medicine approach to education, lifestyle changes, and early assessment in patients with a family history of snoring, sleep apnea, diabetes, and heart disease is warranted. Furthermore, a team-based approach allows for a coordinated precision diagnosis and management of common comorbid chronic illnesses. The significance of sleep disturbances in this population, contributing factors, assessment and diagnostic challenges, common sleep disorders and mechanisms, tailored behavioral and pharmacologic interventions, knowledge gaps, and future research ideas are discussed.

Further Development of P4 Approach to Obstructive Sleep Apnea   379

Allan I. Pack

Obstructive sleep apnea (OSA) is a heterogeneous disorder. Cluster analysis has identified different physiologic subtypes with respect to symptoms. A difference exists in cardiovascular risk from OSA between the 7 subtypes identified. There are

3 basic subtypes replicated in multiple studies: (a) a group where insomnia is the main symptom; (b) an asymptomatic group; (c) a group with marked excessive sleepiness. The symptomatic benefit from treatment with nasal CPAP varies between these 3 subtypes. Data from the Sleep Heart Health Study reveal that the increased risk of cardiovascular disease from OSA occurs only in the excessively sleepy group.

Precision Medicine for Obstructive Sleep Apnea   391

Matthew Light, Robert L. Owens, Christopher N. Schmickl, and Atul Malhotra

Increasingly, obstructive sleep apnea treatment is being recognized as amenable to a precision medicine approach. Many pathophysiologic mechanisms (endotypes) beyond anatomic compromise have now been identified and are readily determined during polysomnography, although randomized controlled trials of endotype-specific therapies are needed. Research indicates that endotypes may also be important in predicting both adherence to therapy and disease consequences (phenotypes). Biomarker discovery and Big Data approaches derived from wearable technology are areas of active investigation and may allow more robust conclusions to be drawn over time, such that patients may soon fully realize the benefits from fresh insights into sleep science.

Precision Medicine for Sleep Loss and Fatigue Management   399

Luis E. Pichard, Guido Simonelli, Lindsay Schwartz, Thomas J. Balkin, and Steven Hursh

Sleep loss is a widespread phenomenon and a public health threat. Sleep disorders, medical conditions, lifestyles, and occupational factors all contribute to insufficient sleep. Regardless of the underlying cause, insufficient sleep has well-defined consequences and the severity of said consequences partially influenced by individual characteristics. It is here where precision medicine needs to understand and define sleep insufficiency in hopes for personalizing medical approach to improve patient outcomes. Following a discussion on causes and consequences of sleep loss, this article discusses tools for assessing sleep sufficiency, mitigating strategies to sleep loss, and sleep loss in the context of fatigue management.

Preface

Precision Medicine in the Field of Sleep Medicine: Early Days

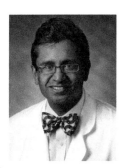

Susheel P. Patil, MD, PhD
Editor

The term "precision medicine" has gained popularity in recent years, particularly when the Obama administration announced its "Precision Medicine Initiative" in 2015, which included focused investments in a national research cohort, identifying genetic drivers in cancer, and modernizing the regulatory landscape to support such research while maintaining privacy.[1]

The National Research Council[2] defined precision medicine as:

> ... the tailoring of medical treatment to the individual characteristics of each patient. It does not literally mean the creation of drugs or medical devices that are unique to a patient, but rather the ability to classify individuals into subpopulations that differ in their susceptibility to a particular disease, in the biology and/or prognosis of those diseases they may develop, or in their response to a specific treatment. Preventive or therapeutic interventions can then be concentrated on those who will benefit, sparing expense and side effects for those who will not. Although the term "personalized medicine" is also used to convey this meaning, that term is sometimes misinterpreted as implying that unique treatments can be designed for each individual.

Much of the focus has been on creating large-scale data sets in areas such as cancer on which big data analytics might be applied to gain insights into different disease phenotypes or phenotype-based responses to treatment. The field of sleep medicine is arguably in the beginning stages of utilizing such an approach to tailor treatments for patients. Some areas of sleep medicine such as obstructive sleep apnea have potential tools[3,4] that can be used as part of a strategy for "deep phenotyping"[5] of patients that needs to be implemented to address precision medicine–related questions. Similarly, areas such as chronic insomnia, individual responses to sleep restriction, and restless legs syndrome show potential promise for applying precision medicine approaches with the identification of genetic markers and application of our understanding of the pharmacogenetics of commonly used medications in sleep medicine. Other areas of sleep medicine, such as idiopathic hypersomnia or some parasomnias, are possibly at an earlier stage for application of precision medicine given the rarity of these disorders.

In this issue of *Sleep Medicine Clinics* entitled, "Precision Sleep Medicine," a collection of articles has been assembled, written by distinguished experts, that address where our field currently is with respect to precision medicine principles for many sleep disorders. Regrettably a few important areas are absent from this issue, which should not be construed as precision medicine approaches that are absent in these areas. I

Sleep Med Clin 14 (2019) xiii–xiv
https://doi.org/10.1016/j.jsmc.2019.06.001
1556-407X/19/© 2019 Published by Elsevier Inc.

would like to thank the contributors to this issue who have created content that should be stimulating to readers and help inform continued discussions of precision medicine within the field of sleep medicine.

Susheel P. Patil, MD, PhD
Division of Pulmonary and
Critical Care Medicine
Johns Hopkins Sleep Disorders Center
Asthma and Allergy Center
5501 Hopkins Bayview Circle
Room 4B.50
Baltimore, MD 21224, USA

E-mail address:
spatil@jhmi.edu

REFERENCES

1. Fact Sheet: President Obama's Precision Medicine Initiative. The Obama White House Web site. January 30, 2015. Available at: https://obamawhitehouse archives.gov/the-press-office/2015/01/30/fact-sheet-president-obama-s-precision-medicine-initiative. Accessed June 3, 2019.

2. Committee on a Framework for Development a New Taxonomy of Disease. National Research Council of the National Academy of Science. Toward precision medicine: building a knowledge network for biomedical research and a new taxonomy of disease. National Academies Press; 2011. Available at: http://www.nap.edu/catalog.php?record_id=13284. Accessed June 3, 2019.

3. Eckert DJ, White DP, Jordan AS, et al. Defining phenotypic causes of obstructive sleep apnea. Identification of novel therapeutic targets. Am J Respir Crit Care Med 2013;188(8):996–1004.

4. Ye L, Pien GW, Ratcliffe SJ, et al. The different clinical faces of obstructive sleep apnoea: a cluster analysis. Eur Respir J 2014;44(6):1600–7.

5. König IR, Fuchs O, Hansen G, et al. What is precision medicine? Eur Resp J 2017;50(4):1–12.

Precision Medicine for Insomnia

Elaine Boland, PhD[a,b], Jennifer Goldschmied, PhD[a], Matthew S. Kayser, MD, PhD[a], Philip R. Gehrman, PhD[a,b],*

KEYWORDS

- Insomnia • CBT-I • Behavioral treatment • Pharmacotherapy • Precision medicine
- Sleep disturbance • Case conceptualization

KEY POINTS

- Insomnia is prevalent in the United States and warrants targeted treatment.
- Cognitive behavioral therapy for insomnia is the front-line treatment of choice for adults with chronic insomnia and is easily delivered in a personalized approach.
- Pharmacotherapeutic options are also effective, but providers must consider individual factors when making decisions about which medications are most appropriate.
- Careful consideration of the individual's symptoms can help providers choose between pharmacotherapy and behavioral treatment to enhance delivery of precision medicine.

INTRODUCTION

Although sleep apnea is the sleep disorder most commonly encountered in sleep medicine clinics, insomnia is much more common in the general population. Insomnia disorder occurs in 10% to 15% of the US population, whereas symptoms of insomnia that may not meet full diagnostic criteria affect another 25% to 35%.[1] Collectively this means that one-third to one-half of individuals struggle with insomnia on at least an occasional basis. The public health impact of insomnia is substantial, with one report citing it as among the top 10 neuropsychiatric causes of burden worldwide.[2] The daytime effects of insomnia include irritability, fatigue, difficulty with memory and concentration, tiredness, and low motivation.[3] Long term, insomnia is associated with increased risk of a range of poor health indicators, including new-onset mental health disorders and cardiovascular disease.[4,5] As such, there is a critical need for more targeted treatment of insomnia.

However, effective treatments exist. The 2 main treatment modalities with demonstrated efficacy are pharmacotherapy and cognitive behavioral therapy for insomnia (CBT-I). Both have been rigorously investigated and supported by a large body of empirical research and are considered treatments that work. There are several good reviews and meta-analyses summarizing the available evidence,[6–8] which are not discussed here. Instead, the focus is on the question of what works for whom. Such is the task of precision medicine, determining which treatments should be used with individual patients. Note that there are several other treatment options that have been reported, but

Disclosure: The authors have no disclosures to report.

Funding: Writing of this article was supported by the Department of Veterans Affairs CSR&D, IK2-CX001501 (Boland). The content is solely the responsibility of the authors and does not necessarily represent the official views of the National Institutes of Health or the US Government.

[a] Department of Psychiatry, Perelman School of Medicine of the University of Pennsylvania, 3535 Market Street, Suite 670, Philadelphia, PA 19104, USA; [b] Michael J. Crescenz VA Medical Center, MIRECC, 2nd Floor, B229 3900 Woodland Ave., Philadelphia, PA 19104, USA

* Corresponding author. Department of Psychiatry, University of Pennsylvania, 3535 Market Street, Suite 670, Philadelphia, PA 19104.

E-mail address: gehrman@upenn.edu

sleep.theclinics.com

most consist of a single or small number of studies and a few well-controlled, randomized trials. As such, they are not the focus of this article. The goal instead is to provide guidance on the selection of insomnia treatment of individual patients. It is important to keep in mind that there are very few empirical studies on precision medicine for insomnia. Much of what is discussed is based on extrapolation of the existing literature and clinical experience. Research studies are needed to test many of the assertions that are made.

COGNITIVE BEHAVIORAL THERAPY FOR INSOMNIA

Since its development, CBT-I has achieved gold-standard status as an insomnia treatment, and, because of its limited likelihood of side effects, has been recommended by the American College of Physicians as the first-line treatment of adults with chronic insomnia.[9] CBT-I has been described in great detail elsewhere,[10] but a short overview is provided here (**Table 1**). CBT-I is a short-term (typically 6–8 sessions) behavioral treatment of insomnia that aims to reduce or eliminate conditioned hyperarousal to the sleeping environment, reduce sleep effort, address sleep-related cognitive distortions, improve sleep hygiene, and as a result improve sleep duration and efficiency. These goals are accomplished through a combination of stimulus control strategies, time-in-bed restriction (ie, sleep-restriction therapy), and cognitive restructuring of dysfunctional beliefs about sleep. Stimulus-control strategies are intended to regularize the sleep/wake cycle and reduce conditioned hyperarousal, and include techniques such as getting out of bed when not sleeping, using the bed only for sleep or sexual activity, avoiding daytime napping, and reducing/eliminating worry in bed. Sleep restriction, developed by Arthur Spielman,[11] is intended to improve sleep efficiency by reducing midsleep awakenings. This improvement is achieved by limiting time in bed to the average amount of sleep per night over the course of a week. For example, an individual who averages 6 hours of sleep per night would be given a 6-hour time-in-bed window. Individuals typically experience a transient increase in sleepiness, but afterward can experience a significant reduction in time spent awake in the middle of the night. Once sleep efficiency, or the ratio of time spent awake versus the time spent in bed, achieves at least 85%, the time-in-bed window is gradually lengthened (ie, 15 minutes at a time) until sleep needs are met and sleep efficiency remains in the acceptable range. Distorted beliefs about sleep are restructured using conventional cognitive behavioral therapy techniques, such as thought challenging and debunking common myths about sleep. Throughout treatment, sleep diaries are used to track subjective changes in treatment targets, such as onset latency, wake after sleep onset, regularity of bed/wake times, sleep efficiency, and duration.

One of the strengths of CBT-I that may be associated with its efficacy rate of approximately 80%[6,7] is its ability to be tailored to patients' as well as providers' needs. For example, CBT-I can be delivered in individual or group formats, both in person or via telehealth, with studies supporting efficacy in all modalities.[12,13] In a group format, CBT-I is typically delivered via a fixed approach that establishes a topic/theme for each session in a manualized fashion. For example, session 1

Table 1
Goals of cognitive behavioral therapy for insomnia and associated treatment approaches

Goal	Approach	Key Points
Reduction or elimination of conditioned hyperarousal to the bed/bedroom	Stimulus control	• Use the bed only for sleeping • Do not worry, plan, and so forth in bed • Get out of bed when not sleeping
Reduce sleep effort	Stimulus control	• Go to bed only when sleepy • Get out of bed when not sleeping
Address negative beliefs about sleep that may perpetuate insomnia	Cognitive restructuring	• Identify dysfunctional beliefs about sleep • Provide psychoeducation about myths vs facts about sleep • Challenge dysfunctional thoughts about sleep and generate more rational cognitions
Eliminate behaviors that may get in the way of healthy sleep	Promote sleep hygiene	• Limit caffeine after noon • Limit alcohol • Keep bedroom quiet, dark, and cool • Exercise regularly but not right before bed

would consist of psychoeducation about sleep and insomnia and an introduction to stimulus control strategies. Session 2 might continue stimulus control strategies, and introduce sleep restriction therapy. Session 3 would address cognitive restructuring, and so on.

An advantage of this fixed approach is that all components of CBT-I are covered in a fixed 6-week to 8-week schedule that may be most beneficial for clinics or providers with limited space or time for individual sessions. However, a drawback is that all individuals in the group may have insomnia but their symptom presentations and routines may differ widely, meaning that some sessions may be more or less applicable to one patient versus another. This drawback can be overcome in individual treatment, which is more amenable to a case conceptualization approach that allows the clinician to better match the treatment to the individual's presenting problem. Case conceptualization helps clinicians identify the factors that are most connected to the patient's insomnia, including factors that affect sleep regulation (ie, the underlying biological clock, hyperarousal, sleep drive/propensity); substances such as alcohol, caffeine, nicotine, and illicit drugs or prescription medications; and medical/psychiatric comorbidities.[14] Often, these factors are interrelated, so a solid understanding of how the individual's insomnia may have developed and how these factors contributed to and/or perpetuate the disorder are critical to developing an effective tailored treatment plan.

As an example, consider a man in his mid-30s who reports getting about 6 hours of choppy sleep each night. He has generally healthy sleep hygiene, (ie, does not watch television in bed, does not consume caffeine late in the day, has a regular bedtime routine, and tends to get in and out of bed at approximately the same time each day) but he spends about an hour each night in bed thinking about the next days' obligations, worrying about his job, and trying to problem solve before tomorrow arrives. He then wakes up about twice each night, taking at least a half hour to get back to sleep because of thinking about how much time there is left to sleep before having to get out of bed for work. The insomnia began approximately 6 months ago, which coincided with a promotion at work and increases in his stress, but before that time he had no problems with sleep. He is otherwise physically and psychiatrically healthy, with no notable medical or mental health treatment history.

Following the case conceptualization approach, it can be hypothesized that the individual's insomnia was precipitated by an increase in stress from his new job. Given fairly healthy sleep hygiene and routine regularity, a clinician might choose to begin with strategies that reduce the patient's hyperarousal at night. For example, generating a "buffer zone" before bed when the individual engages in relaxing activities and gives himself some space between his hectic day and bedtime might be emphasized, and/or the technique of scheduling a "worry time," or a fixed time each day when he allows himself to engage in work-related worry, next-day planning, and so forth. Stimulus control strategies of getting out of bed when not sleeping may also be used to reduce conditioned hyperarousal to his bed. Given that his sleep is disrupted, a 6-hour time-in-bed window may also be established to improve quality and efficiency of sleep, gradually extending that window as sleep improves. The case conceptualization approach allows providers to select the most important issues in an individual's insomnia presentation and address them first, which may increase effectiveness as well as patient adherence and buy-in.

Certain strategies within CBT-I can also be customized to individuals' needs, preferences, and limitations (**Table 2**). For example, the concept of sleep restriction can be anxiety provoking, and individuals who already experience increased levels of hyperarousal and worry about sleep may be more reluctant to engage in this practice. For those individuals, sleep compression[15] may be a more palatable option. As opposed to the immediate reduction of time in bed to match time spent asleep, sleep compression is a more gradual restriction of time in bed. Methods of administering sleep compression can vary, but a general recommendation is to begin with a time-in-bed window of 7.5 hours and then work gradually toward the total sleep window in half-hour increments each week. Another example is that some individuals may have mobility issues that limit the application of stimulus control strategies (eg, getting out of bed in the middle of the night when not sleeping). Individuals who are at a greater risk for falls, or those who are unable to easily get in and out of bed, may struggle with this strategy, and it may be risky. A strategy called countercontrol, which is a variant of stimulus control, may be the better option for these individuals. In countercontrol, rather than getting out of bed when unable to sleep, the individual is asked to sit up in bed, read, or do some other type of relaxing activity rather than continue to lie down and struggle to get back to sleep.

Although CBT-I is an effective, evidence-based treatment of insomnia, some care must be taken to determine the patient's appropriateness for

Table 2
Personalization of traditional cognitive behavioral therapy for insomnia approaches

Obstacle to Traditional Administration	Option for Personalization
Anxiety about the drastic change to time in bed that comes with sleep restriction	Sleep compression; gradually decrease the time-in-bed window over the course of several weeks rather than all at once
Medical condition that places individual at risk for falls	Countercontrol; rather than advise individuals to get out of bed when not sleeping, have them sit upright in bed and avoid a sleeping position
Comorbid diagnosis of: • Bipolar disorder • Seizures • Untreated sleep apnea with excessive daytime sleepiness	Avoid sleep restriction; continue to follow other CBT-I strategies with a focus on regularizing sleep/wake schedules
The individual has PTSD and is participating in PE therapy	Consider treating insomnia before PE, or delaying until after PE is completed
Severe drug or alcohol dependence	Address substance issues first and then revisit CBT-I when the individual is in remission

Abbreviations: PE, prolonged exposure; PTSD, posttraumatic stress disorder.

the treatment, because components of CBT-I, namely sleep restriction, are contraindicated in the context of certain medical and psychiatric conditions. For example, sleep loss, even the transient sleep loss associated with sleep restriction, can increase the likelihood of seizures in individuals with seizure disorder, and sleep loss has been associated with onset of manic episodes in individuals with bipolar disorder.[16] In addition, the transient increases in sleepiness that can occur with sleep restriction can be risky in individuals with severe, untreated sleep apnea who already experience excessive daytime sleepiness, and, as such, sleep restriction is generally avoided in those individuals. However, CBT-I lends itself to a modular approach in which components of the treatment can be helpful in reducing insomnia

symptoms even when the full CBT-I package cannot be administered. For example, individuals with bipolar disorder often experience increased irregularity in sleep routines[17] and may benefit from strategies designed to generate a fixed wake time. Depending on the individual's case presentation, other stimulus control strategies may also be beneficial, depending on the degree of hyperarousal experienced.

In addition, CBT-I can be part of personalizing insomnia treatment of individuals with overarching medical or mental health concerns. For example, insomnia is often comorbid with several psychiatric disorders, including posttraumatic stress disorder (PTSD), depression, anxiety, and substance abuse.[18] It is also common among individuals with chronic pain, and may develop as a consequence of medical disorders or treatment (ie, frequent nighttime urination from prostate enlargement, blood pressure pills, or type II diabetes). In these cases, insomnia is often interconnected with the co-occurring disorder, and some care should be taken to determine whether insomnia can be addressed concurrently or in a stepped-care format. For example, one of the leading evidence-based treatments for PTSD is prolonged exposure (PE), a treatment that can be difficult for patients with a significant amount of homework after sessions. In general, it is not advisable to conduct CBT-I concurrently with PE because of the heavy behavioral requirements of both treatments. However, there is some emerging evidence that 6 sessions of CBT-I administered before PE can improve PTSD outcomes.[19] Thus, a stepped-care model in which insomnia is addressed before PTSD symptoms may be an effective treatment plan for individuals who struggle with significant sleep disturbance in the context of PTSD.

In contrast, certain disorders may affect the effectiveness of CBT-I and should be addressed before engaging fully in this form of insomnia treatment. For example, insomnia is often present in individuals with alcohol dependence[20]; many individuals use alcohol as a means of self-medicating symptoms of sleep disturbance. However, in individuals addicted to and dependent on alcohol, treatment of the underlying addiction and its associated health concerns is the advisable first step. It is difficult, if not impossible, to fully adhere to CBT-I strategies while continuing to abuse alcohol, and the health and safety risks associated with alcohol abuse warrant more immediate attention. However, insomnia often lingers once sobriety is achieved,[21] and CBT-I may be an effective option once consistent abstinence has been achieved.[22]

Overall, CBT-I is a highly customizable treatment, allowing clinicians to tailor strategies to their patients' unique needs. However, although CBT-I is the recommended first-line treatment of adults with chronic insomnia, there are still patients for whom CBT-I is not the best option. In other cases, patients may lack access to providers trained in CBT-I. In these cases, pharmacotherapy remains an effective treatment option for insomnia.

PHARMACOTHERAPY

When it comes to pharmacotherapy for insomnia, there are several medications to choose from. However, this can make the choice of medication for an individual patient daunting. How should clinicians select the best medication based on patient characteristics? The options for pharmacotherapy include both US Food and Drug Administration–approved sedative hypnotics and off-label use of medications with sedating side effects. The main categories of medications used for insomnia include non–benzodiazepine receptor antagonists (non-BZRAs), benzodiazepines, sedating antidepressants, melatonin receptor agonists, antihistamines, and dual orexin receptor antagonists (see Ref.[23] for more detailed coverage of a pharmacologic options).

Insomnia is often categorized as difficulty with falling asleep at the beginning of the sleep period (sleep-onset insomnia), waking up in the middle of the night with difficulty returning to sleep (sleep-maintenance insomnia), or waking up earlier than desired in the morning and being unable to get back to sleep (early-morning awakenings). When selecting a medication, one of the most important factors to consider is the half-life, which for sleep medication can range from 1.5 hours for zaleplon to more than 24 hours for some benzodiazepines. The longer the half-life, the greater the likelihood that the patient will be able to sleep through the night. The primary disadvantage of a longer half-life is the potential for next-day sedation: patients may be able to sleep well at night but have difficulty waking up in the morning, and may not feel fully awake for several hours; some go as far as to state that the cure is worse than the problem. The potential for oversedation can be a safety concern, because patients who drive or operate machinery in the morning may be impaired. Short-acting medications are less likely to cause grogginess the next day, but patients sometimes report improved sleep-onset latency with middle-of-the-night awakenings and difficulty sleeping the rest of the night. For patients with primarily sleep-onset insomnia, a short-acting medication may be sufficient to help them fall asleep without awakenings for the rest of the night. If early-morning awakenings are present, a longer-acting medication may be needed. The proportion of the night affected can guide the selection of the appropriate medication. A limitation of this approach is that, for most patients, insomnia is not limited to 1 portion of the night.[24] In addition, the presenting pattern can change over time, making for a moving target.

In the context of precision medicine for insomnia, another important factor to take into consideration is comorbid disorders, in particular psychiatric comorbidities. As described earlier, roughly 80% of patients with insomnia have 1 or more comorbidities that could affect sleep and wakefulness.[18] In the selection of a sleep medication, there is the opportunity to select an agent that could improve both insomnia and 1 or more comorbidities. For example, insomnia is frequently comorbid with anxiety disorders.[25] Although there is reason to be cautious in the use of benzodiazepines for the treatment of insomnia or anxiety, they may be a good short-term option for patients with significant insomnia and anxiety given the anxiolytic effects of this class of medication. Depression is another disorder that commonly co-occurs with insomnia disorder. Sedating antidepressants such as mirtazapine can be useful for both the insomnia and the depression. Trazodone is one of the most commonly used medications for sleep, even though it is approved as an antidepressant, and it is rarely used any more for depression. It is important to keep in mind that some antidepressant medications, such as selective serotonin reuptake inhibitors, can cause or worsen insomnia as a side effect and so should be used cautiously in patients with both conditions. An alternative to selecting a dual-use medication is to use one medication for the treatment of insomnia and another for the psychiatric comorbidity, but this polypharmacy approach increases the risk of side effects and drug-drug interactions.

COGNITIVE BEHAVIORAL THERAPY FOR INSOMNIA VERSUS PHARMACOTHERAPY

As discussed earlier, CBT-I and pharmacologic treatments can both confer significant benefit to individuals experiencing symptoms of insomnia. In order to quantify these benefits, researchers have tried to take a big-picture approach by summarizing the full scope of the studies that have sought to directly assess treatment outcomes, including systematic reviews and meta-analyses. For example, in their systematic review, Mitchell and colleagues[8] report that benzodiazepine receptor agonists (BZRAs) showed moderate efficacy, while noting that pharmacologic approaches are the most common treatment of insomnia. They also report that the randomized clinical trials conducted to date on the effectiveness of CBT-I reveal that CBT-I is as effective as hypnotics for the treatment of insomnia, and confers greater long-term benefits.

In a similar fashion, Riemann and Perlis[26] examined the meta-analytical evidence of both BZRAs and CBT-I. With regard to BZRAs, they reviewed 4 meta-analyses and concluded that although the 4 studies were not consistent, it was clear that the use of BZRAs was associated with acute clinical improvement. However, they did note that the meta-analytical evidence indicated that BZRAs may not be an appropriate first-line choice for older adults. Concerning the effectiveness of psychological and behavioral treatments, Riemann and Perlis[26] reviewed 5 meta-analyses and determined that the use of behavioral treatments was associated with robust clinical improvements and long-term gains, with no limitation for use with older adults. In addition, although they state that there is little comparative research on the use of BZRAs versus CBT-I, they were able to review 5 studies and 1 meta-analysis that directly compared behavioral treatments with pharmacotherapy. Similar to Mitchell and colleagues,[8] they concluded that behavioral treatments like CBT-I are equally effective during active treatment and sustain longer-term gains than pharmacotherapy.

From this body of research, it can be seen that, in general, CBT-I has durable treatment effects that result from a short treatment course of approximately 4 to 8 sessions. In contrast, CBT-I is not a fast-acting treatment, and individuals engaging in CBT-I may not begin to see benefit until session 3 to 4, which may take several weeks. Hypnotics work much more quickly, with improvements in sleep-onset latency and wake after sleep onset in as little as 1 night. However, there are few data on the safety or efficacy of long-term use of hypnotics, which is crucially important because the effects of hypnotics do not persist past the active treatment period, and long-term use may be associated with drug tolerance, dependence, rapid eye movement rebound, insomnia rebound, and daytime impairments caused by morning somnolence. Because the emerging evidence continues to suggest that CBT-I is a superior treatment of insomnia compared with pharmacotherapy, the American College of Physicians (ACP) released a statement in 2016 recommending that CBT-I be the initial treatment choice for chronic insomnia.[9]

The ACP recommendation was especially strong with regard to older adults because morning somnolence is an importance concern in this group because of heightened fall risk. CBT-I has also been indicated as the preferred treatment of other groups. For example, by both systematic review and meta-analysis, CBT-I has been shown to be an effective treatment of patients with cancer and survivors, improving sleep efficiency and self-reported insomnia severity.[27,28] Both studies strongly supported a recommendation for CBT-I for patients with cancer and survivors based on all available evidence. Although there have been no comparative studies of hypnotics versus CBT-I in this population, 1 review of the existing literature concluded that, because of the risk profile of long-term hypnotic use, CBT-I is the preferred treatment of this group.[29] In addition, when considering comorbid psychiatric illness like major depressive disorder (MDD), CBT-I is also considered the favorable treatment. In MDD, symptoms of insomnia are prevalent and associated with worse outcomes, so typical treatment regimens may include an antidepressant coupled with a hypnotic medication.[30] However, they suggest that, because of the risk of drug-drug interactions, and because CBT-I can easily be integrated into an existing psychotherapeutic approach for the treatment of depression, CBT-I should be the first-line approach for the treatment of insomnia in MDD.

In contrast, there are instances when CBT-I may not be a robust enough treatment to reduce symptoms of insomnia. Vgontzas and Fernandez-Mendoza[31] have suggested that insomnia with objectively measured short sleep duration of less than 6 hours is the most biologically severe phenotype of the disorder. They report that this phenotype shows physiologic and emotional hyperarousal that is associated with HPA-axis activation, and increased risk for poor health outcomes such as hypertension and diabetes, and mortality. They suggest that this phenotype may have a biological basis associated with a genetic predisposition or hyperactive physiology that may respond better to biologically based treatments that aim to reduce physiologic arousal, such as hypnotic medications. In support of this hypothesis, Bathgate and colleagues[32] recently showed that individuals with insomnia and objective short sleep duration, as assessed by actigraphy, showed fewer gains from CBT-I than those with normal sleep duration. They qualify these results by highlighting that the study was limited to individuals reporting sleep maintenance complaints, and that the findings may also be related to a floor effect for sleep restriction, because guidelines for treatment recommend a minimum of 5 hours. However, they suggest that

Table 3
Pros and cons of cognitive behavioral therapy for insomnia versus pharmacotherapy

	CBT-I	Pharmacotherapy
Pros	Associated with robust clinical improvement and long-term gains	Use of BZRAs associated with acute clinical improvement
	No limitations for older adults	Fast-acting treatment response
	Longer-term gains compared with pharmacotherapy	—
	Considered the favorable treatment of patients with comorbid conditions (eg, mental health diagnoses; cancer)	—
Cons	Not a fast-acting treatment	BRZAs may not be the most appropriate first-time treatment of older adults
	May not be a robust enough treatment of individuals with insomnia and short sleep duration	No data on safety or efficacy of long-term hypnotic use
	Sleep restriction is associated with initial increase in daytime sleepiness, which can lead to treatment dropout	Risk of dependence, tolerance, REM rebound, insomnia rebound, and daytime impairment

Abbreviation: REM, rapid eye movement.

These results support the need for an alternative treatment strategy for insomnia with objective short sleep duration. In contrast, another study recently showed that CBT-I was as effective in patients with short sleep duration as normal sleep duration.[33] Although this theory has inconsistent support, one potential solution, highlighted by Vgontzas and Fernandez-Mendoza,[31] may be the use of a combination treatment, with both a biological component(ie, hypnotics) and a psychological intervention (ie, CBT-I).

Taken together, the literature seems to converge on suggesting that CBT-I is a better treatment than pharmacotherapy with regard to durability of treatment outcomes and risk of side effects in most patient populations (**Table 3**). In addition, CBT-I has recently been shown to reduce the need for hypnotics among outpatients.[34] However, there remain several considerations that should be taken into account when choosing a treatment strategy for insomnia. CBT-I is not always covered by health insurance, and CBT-I practitioners may not be accessible in all areas. With regard to accessibility, the tide may be shifting, with evidence suggesting that CBT-I delivered by telehealth or using online applications are effective in reducing insomnia symptoms,[12,13,35–37] which would allow CBT-I to be offered in even the most rural areas.

Another important factor in considering treatment with CBT-I is that one of the most effective components of the intervention is sleep restriction,[38] which is associated with an initial increase in daytime sleepiness. A significant increase in subjective daytime sleepiness can lead individuals to drop out of treatment, citing difficulties with daytime functioning. Relatedly, Manber and colleagues[30] suggest that sleep restriction, like sleep deprivation, can also increase individuals' sensitivity to the side effects of other concomitant medications, such as antidepressants, which might likewise lead to treatment failure. Given that the literature has shown positive treatment outcomes for both approaches, individuals with insomnia should be confident that they can effectively manage their symptoms.

REFERENCES

1. Ohayon MM. Epidemiology of insomnia: what we know and what we still need to learn. Sleep Med Rev 2002;6(2):97–111.
2. Collins PY, Patel V, Joestl SS, et al. Grand challenges in global mental health. Nature 2011;475(7354): 27–30.
3. Benca R. Consequences of insomnia and its therapies. J Clin Psychiatry 2001;62:33–8.
4. Baglioni C, Battagliese G, Feige B, et al. Insomnia as a predictor of depression: a meta-analytic evaluation of longitudinal epidemiological studies. J Affect Disord 2011;135(1–3):10–9.
5. Javaheri S, Redline S. Insomnia and risk of cardiovascular disease. Chest 2017;152(2):435–44.
6. Smith MT, Perlis ML, Park A, et al. Comparative meta-analysis of pharmacotherapy and behavior therapy for persistent insomnia. Am J Psychiatry 2002;159(1):5–11.

7. Murtagh DR, Greenwood KM. Identifying effective psychological treatments for insomnia: a meta-analysis. J Consult Clin Psychol 1995;63:79–89.

8. Mitchell MD, Gehrman P, Perlis M, et al. Comparative effectiveness of cognitive behavioral therapy for insomnia: a systematic review. BMC Fam Pract 2012;13:40.

9. Qaseem A, Kansagara D, Forciea MA, et al, Clinical Guidelines Committee of the American College of Physicians. Management of chronic insomnia disorder in adults: a clinical practice guideline from the American College of Physicians. Ann Intern Med 2016;165(2):125–33.

10. Trauer JM, Qian MY, Doyle JS, et al. Cognitive behavioral therapy for chronic insomnia: a systematic review and meta-analysis. Ann Intern Med 2015;163(3):191–204.

11. Spielman AJ, Saskin P, Thorpy MJ. Treatment of chronic insomnia by restriction of time in bed. Sleep 1987;10:45–56.

12. Gehrman P, Shah MT, Miles A, et al. Feasibility of group cognitive behavioral treatment of insomnia delivered by clinical video telehealth. Telemed J E Health 2016;22(12):1041–6.

13. Koffel EA, Koffel JB, Gehrman PR. A meta-analysis of group cognitive behavioral therapy for insomnia. Sleep Med Rev 2015;19:6–16.

14. Manber R, Friedman L, Siebern A, et al. Cognitive behavioral therapy for insomnia in Veterans: therapist manual. Washington, DC: U.S. Department of Veterans Affairs; 2014.

15. Lichstein KL, Riedel BW, Wilson NM, et al. Relaxation and sleep compression for late-life insomnia: a placebo-controlled trial. J Consult Clin Psychol 2001;69(2):227–39.

16. Wehr TA. Sleep loss: a preventable cause of mania and other excited states. J Clin Psychiatry 1989; 50(Suppl):8–16 [discussion: 45–7].

17. Ng TH, Chung KF, Ng TK, et al. Correlates and prognostic relevance of sleep irregularity in inter-episode bipolar disorder. Compr Psychiatry 2016;69:155–62.

18. Buysse DJ, Reynolds CF 3rd, Kupfer DJ, et al. Clinical diagnoses in 216 insomnia patients using the international classification of sleep disorders (ICSD), DSM-IV and ICD-10 categories: a report from the APA/NIMH DSM-IV field trial. Sleep 1994;17(7): 630–7.

19. Colvonen PJ, Drummond SPA, Angkaw AC, et al. Piloting cognitive-behavioral therapy for insomnia integrated with prolonged exposure. Psychol Trauma 2019;11(1):107–13.

20. Chaudhary NS, Kampman KM, Kranzler HR, et al. Insomnia in alcohol dependent subjects is associated with greater psychosocial problem severity. Addict Behav 2015;50:165–72.

21. Brower KJ. Insomnia, alcoholism and relapse. Sleep Med Rev 2003;7(6):523–39.

22. Chakravorty S, Vandrey RG, He S, et al. Sleep management among patients with substance use disorders. Med Clin North Am 2018;102(4):733–43.

23. Frase L, Nissen C, Riemann D, et al. Making sleep easier: pharmacological interventions for insomnia. Expert Opin Pharmacother 2018;19(13):1465–73.

24. Buysse DJ, Finn L, Young T. Onset, remission persistence, and consistency of insomnia symptoms over 10 years: longitudinal results from the Wisconsin Sleep Cohort Study (WSCS). Sleep 2004 27(Supp):A268.

25. Glidewell RN, McPherson Botts E, Orr WC. Insomnia and anxiety: diagnostic and management implications of complex interactions. Sleep Med Clin 2015;10(1):93–9.

26. Riemann D, Perlis ML. The treatments of chronic insomnia: a review of benzodiazepine receptor agonists and psychological and behavioral therapies. Sleep Med Rev 2009;13(3):205–14.

27. Howell D, Oliver TK, Keller-Olaman S, et al. Sleep disturbance in adults with cancer: a systematic review of evidence for best practices in assessment and management for clinical practice. Ann Oncol 2014;25(4):791–800.

28. Johnson JA, Rash JA, Campbell TS, et al. A systematic review and meta-analysis of randomized controlled trials of cognitive behavior therapy for insomnia (CBT-I) in cancer survivors. Sleep Med Rev 2016;27:20–8.

29. Savard J, Morin CM. Insomnia in the context of cancer: a review of a neglected problem. J Clin Oncol 2001;19(3):895–908.

30. Manber R, Buysse DJ, Edinger J, et al. Efficacy of cognitive-behavioral therapy for insomnia combined with antidepressant pharmacotherapy in patients with comorbid depression and insomnia: a randomized controlled trial. J Clin Psychiatry 2016;77(10): e1316–23.

31. Vgontzas AN, Fernandez-Mendoza J. Insomnia with short sleep duration: nosological, diagnostic, and treatment implications. Sleep Med Clin 2013;8(3) 309–22.

32. Bathgate CJ, Edinger JD, Krystal AD. Insomnia patients with objective short sleep duration have a blunted response to cognitive behavioral therapy for insomnia. Sleep 2017;40(1). https://doi.org/10. 1093/sleep/zsw012.

33. Cronlein T, Wetter TC, Rupprecht R, et al. Cognitive behavioral treatment for insomnia is equally effective in insomnia patients with objective short and normal sleep duration. Sleep Med 2018. https://doi.org/10. 1016/j.sleep.2018.10.038.

34. Park KM, Kim TH, Kim WJ, et al. Cognitive behavioral therapy for insomnia reduces hypnotic prescriptions. Psychiatry Investig 2018;15(5):499–504.

35. Lichstein KL, Scogin F, Thomas SJ, et al. Telehealth cognitive behavior therapy for co-occurring

insomnia and depression symptoms in older adults. J Clin Psychol 2013;69(10):1056–65.

36. Holmqvist M, Vincent N, Walsh K. Web- vs. telehealth-based delivery of cognitive behavioral therapy for insomnia: a randomized controlled trial. Sleep Med 2014;15(2):187–95.

37. Espie CA, Kyle SD, Williams C, et al. A randomized, placebo-controlled trial of online cognitive behavioral therapy for chronic insomnia disorder delivered via an automated media-rich web application. Sleep 2012;35(6):769–81.

38. Kyle SD, Aquino MR, Miller CB, et al. Towards standardisation and improved understanding of sleep restriction therapy for insomnia disorder: a systematic examination of CBT-I trial content. Sleep Med Rev 2015;23:83–8.

Internet-Delivered Cognitive Behavioral Therapy for Insomnia
Tailoring Cognitive Behavioral Therapy for Insomnia for Patients with Chronic Insomnia

Tanja van der Zweerde, MSc[a],*, Jaap Lancee, PhD[b,c],
Annemarie Ida Luik, PhD[d], Annemieke van Straten, PhD[a]

KEYWORDS

- Chronic insomnia • Insomnia • Internet • Cognitive behavioral therapy (CBT)
- CBT for Insomnia (CBTI) • Online psychological treatment • Tailoring treatment

KEY POINTS

- Insomnia is an important public health issue with high prevalence, disease burden, and economic costs. Insomnia is preferably treated with cognitive behavioral therapy (CBTI).
- Both face-to-face and Internet-delivered CBT for Insomnia (I-CBTI) are evidence-based effective treatments.
- I-CBTI has yet to reach its full potential in both scope and scale. More developments toward improved effectiveness could further improve I-CBTI.
- I-CBTI can be successfully offered to a wide and varied range of insomnia sufferers and is suggested to be effective irrespective of demographic variation or baseline severity.
- Research should focus on working mechanisms and moderators of effects, aimed at implementation of tailored Internet treatments to successfully treat more people.

PRECISION MEDICINE FOR INSOMNIA DISORDER

Insomnia is a common mental disorder, characterized by complaints of dissatisfaction with sleep quantity, sleep quality, or both. Persons with insomnia suffer from these symptoms 3 or more nights per week, for at least 3 months, which results in significant distress or impaired daytime functioning (*Diagnostic and Statistical Manual of Mental Disorders, 5th Edition: DSM-5*[1]; for full criteria see **Table 1**). Approximately one-third of the population suffers from occasional insomnia symptoms, whereas approximately 7% to 10% fit

Disclosure Statement: The online cognitive behavioral therapy for insomnia program, i-Sleep, was developed at the VU University Amsterdam by Annemieke van Straten and further developed in collaboration with Jaap Lancee (University of Amsterdam) and T. van der Zweerde (VU University). The authors have no commercial interest in this program. Annemarie Luik has previously worked in a position funded by Big Health Inc. (Sleepio); she currently has no commercial or financial interest in Big Health Inc.
[a] Department of Clinical Psychology, EMGO Institute for Health and Care Research, VU University, Van der Boechorststraat 7, Amsterdam 1081 BT, the Netherlands; [b] Department of Clinical Psychology, University of Amsterdam, Nieuwe Achtergracht 129, Amsterdam 1018 WS, the Netherlands; [c] PsyQ Amsterdam, Amsterdam, the Netherlands; [d] Department of Epidemiology, Erasmus MC University Medical Center, Dr. Molewaterplein 40, Rotterdam 3015 GD, the Netherlands
* Corresponding author.
E-mail address: t.vander.zweerde@vu.nl

Sleep Med Clin 14 (2019) 301–315
https://doi.org/10.1016/j.jsmc.2019.04.002

Table 1
DSM-5 and ICSD-3 diagnosis of insomnia disorder

Classification System	Duration	Frequency	Sleep Complaints
DSM-5	≥3 mo	≥3 nights per week	Difficulty initiating sleep, maintaining sleep, and/or early morning awakening with inability to return to sleep despite adequate opportunity for sleep.
			Resulting in significant impairment of daytime functioning and/or significant distress.
			Not better explained by another sleep-wake disorder, physiologic effects of substances or coexistent conditions.
ICSD-3	≥3 mo	≥3 nights per week	Difficulty initiating sleep, maintaining sleep, waking up earlier than desired, resistance to going to bed at appropriate time, and/or difficulty sleeping without intervention.
			Fatigue/malaise, impaired attention/concentration/memory, impaired performance (social, familial, occupational, or academic), mood disturbance/irritability, daytime sleepiness, behavioral problems (eg, hyperactivity, impulsivity, or aggression), reduced motivation/energy/initiative, proneness to judgment errors or to physical accidents, and/or concerns about or dissatisfaction with sleep.
			Reported sleep-wake complaints cannot be explained purely by inadequate opportunity or circumstance for sleep: enough time has been allotted for sleep and the environment is safe, dark, quiet, and comfortable.
			Sleep-wake difficulty is not better explained by another sleep disorder (intoxication and acute withdrawal are ruled out).

Abbreviations: DSM-5, diagnostic and statistical manual of mental disorders, 5th Edition: DSM-5; ICSD-3, international classification of sleep disorders. Third Edition.

clinical criteria for an insomnia diagnosis.[2,3] People typically suffer from insomnia for multiple years[3] before diagnosis. Insomnia also increases the risk for other mental and physical health problems, and persons with insomnia often develop comorbid mental health problems, such as depression or anxiety.[4–6] The economic burden of insomnia is considerable: poor sleepers cost society up to 10 times as much as good sleepers.[7,8] The high prevalence, costs, burden, and risk of insomnia warrant efficacious treatment. Precision medicine offers the potential to realize the best use of limited time and resources in (mental) health care. Internet-delivered therapy can facilitate a precision medicine approach, as components, intensity, order, reminders, and guidance can be tailored to suit the specific needs of the patient, but at the same time needs fewer resources than face-to-face solutions for precision medicine.

COGNITIVE BEHAVIORAL THERAPY FOR INSOMNIA

Currently, many people seeking help for insomnia are prescribed a pharmacologic treatment, mostly benzodiazepines or benzodiazepine receptor agonists (the so-called "Z-drugs": zolpidem, zopiclone, zaleplon[9]). As short-term treatment, pharmacotherapies are effective in relieving insomnia[10–12]; however, pharmacotherapy has negative side effects,

such as headaches, drowsiness and dizziness can alter sleep microstructure, and potentially leads to dependency and addiction when used long-term.[11–13] When a person quits medication, the person can also suffer from rebound effects.[14] Furthermore, the evidence for longer-term effects of pharmacotherapies is limited.[15–17] Despite these concerns, in the United States, use of prescription sleep aids has increased in recent years.[10] Other psychoactive medications such as antidepressants or antipsychotics are also used to treat insomnia even though their effectiveness has not adequately been demonstrated in clinical trials.[18]

Fortunately, evidence-based alternatives to pharmacotherapy for persons with insomnia are available. Since the 1990s, a collection of different treatment components (educational, behavioral, and cognitive) has been offered as a combined treatment: cognitive behavioral therapy for insomnia (CBTI). An overview of the different components of CBTI is listed in **Table 2**.[21]

Multiple reviews have concluded that CBTI is effective and has effects that last longer than those of pharmacologic treatments for insomnia. As a result, CBTI has a substantial evidence base for the treatment of insomnia.[16,22–29] Large posttreatment effects are reported on insomnia severity (Hedges $'g = 0.98$), self-rated sleep efficiency ($g = 0.71$) and sleep quality ($g = 0.65^{29}$). A recent meta-analysis[30] demonstrated that CBTI has

Table 2
Core cognitive behavioral therapy for insomnia components

Component	Content
Psycho-education	Information about the process and function of normal and disturbed sleep.
Sleep hygiene and lifestyle advice	Information about a healthy lifestyle that can promote sleep (eg, low caffeine and alcohol intake), about behaviors and habits that hinder sleep, about adjustments that can be made to improve their sleep (eg, a suitable bedroom and bedtime routine). Fixed hours are set for bed and rising times aiming to stabilize the circadian rhythm.
Stimulus control	Person's associations between bed and sleep are reaffirmed by advice to get out of bed when awake >15 min, and only go back to bed when sleepy. The bed is to be used for sleep and sexual activity only.
Sleep restriction therapy	Person's time in bed is restricted to the average time a patient slept the past week (typically with a minimum of 5 hours). This heightens the homeostatic sleep drive (ie, patients are more tired), making them fall asleep easier and strengthens the bed-sleep association. When this results in less fragmented sleep, the sleep window is elongated slowly (see Refs.[19,20]).
Relaxation techniques	Different relaxation and breathing exercises are used to teach patients to unwind and take more breaks during the day, for example, progressive muscle relaxation or meditation exercises.
Cognitive restructuring	Persons identify and challenge misconceptions (such as "I have to sleep 8 h a night") and worries that keep them awake. These might be related to sleep or to other non–sleep-related issues. Unhelpful thoughts are unpacked and challenged using cognitive techniques, such as gathering evidence for and against a certain belief or statement, and gathering evidence for a more helpful alternative.

positive long-term effects that last up to a year, showing an effect of clinically significant magnitude. Because of these favorable effects, international guidelines recommend CBTI as a first-line treatment rather than prescribing medication, or combining the 2 modalities if necessary.[31,32]

Online Cognitive Behavioral Therapy for Insomnia

Although CBTI is recommended therapy for insomnia, many patients with insomnia do not receive CBTI. Several important reasons for this discrepancy can be identified. First, estimates are that only 50% of persons with insomnia actively seek help.[33] Second, given the high prevalence of insomnia[2] and the relatively small number of trained CBTI therapists, there is a discrepancy between the demand for treatment and available resources. Moreover, health care budgets are not sufficient to provide face-to-face CBT to everyone, even if therapists were available.

Third, general practitioners (GPs), often the first point of contact for persons with insomnia who seek treatment, rarely refer to psychological treatments for insomnia.[34]

As a potential solution to some of these issues CBTI could be offered in an online format (I-CBTI). Because I-CBTI requires less therapist input than face-to-face therapy, the same number of therapists can treat many more people. Furthermore, I-CBTI might be less stigmatizing and more easily accessible to patients. Going to a health care professional, such as a GP, is required in most cases to obtain access to online treatment, but patients may nonetheless regard this as a smaller and more easily accomplished step than being referred to mental health care facilities for help.

CBTI in an online format is similar to CBTI delivered face-to-face, containing mostly the same elements in the same order. Typically, I-CBTI is offered through secured Web sites that include informative texts, videos, graphs, and illustrations.

Participants provide information to the program via (interactive) questionnaires and a sleep diary. Many variations of I-CBTI exist, including variations that (1) use a mix of face-to-face sessions and I-CBTI, (2) use support and feedback from a health care professional, and (3) use fully automated support and feedback, either personalized or not. In most treatments, the number of sessions and their order is fixed, but some programs have opt-in elements in which participants can select components that they feel are relevant for them,[35] or provide a mix of fixed and optional components.[36]

EFFICACY OF INTERNET-DELIVERED COGNITIVE BEHAVIORAL THERAPY FOR INSOMNIA

In 2004, Ström and colleagues[37] published the first randomized controlled study investigating Internet-based treatment for insomnia. Since then, many more studies and digital programs for insomnia have been developed. To our knowledge, 13 different I-CBTI programs have been studied in a randomized controlled trial (Refs.[35–49]; **Table 3**), of which most programs were developed for adults except 1 program for adolescents.[49] Although the number of online treatments for insomnia is expected to continue to grow rapidly, only a small percentage has been evidence-based so far, leaving many more programs without any evidence base accompanied by unknown efficacy and risks, potentially even causing harm.

GUIDANCE IN ONLINE COGNITIVE BEHAVIORAL THERAPY FOR INSOMNIA PROGRAMS

Most programs offer at least some form of therapeutic guidance, either automated or by a therapist, that is, human feedback. Common elements are feedback on sleep diaries that a person keeps, as well as motivational messages to help participants adhere to the program, and providing additional instructions and explanations when necessary. Participants usually receive online feedback and motivational support for every session they complete. Providing human feedback takes an estimated 15 to 30 minutes per online participant per session and can be provided by psychologists, other health care professionals, or by clinical psychology students.[36,52,54,57] Automated feedback also is used.[35,39,48] Extensive programming ensures that participants receive tailored messages suited to their situation and sleep patterns.

Research on online treatments for other psychological disorders reports that support promotes adherence and increases effects[58]; however, only 2 studies have investigated these effects in online insomnia treatment. Both report that support, even if it is very limited, improves effectiveness.[59,60] More research is needed to identify the optimal form and dosage of support. If I-CBTI is to offer a true alternative to pharmacotherapy and be implemented on a large scale, personal (online) support or guidance could present a challenge. Current and future developments not yet applied to I-CBTI could be used to enhance automated support and guidance, for example, by using avatars and/or artificial intelligence.

EFFECTS OF INTERNET-DELIVERED COGNITIVE BEHAVIORAL THERAPY FOR INSOMNIA
Effects on Insomnia of Internet-Delivered Cognitive Behavioral Therapy for Insomnia

Overall, I-CBTI is effective and effect sizes seem in the same range as those of face-to-face treatments,[61] in line with research in, for example, Internet treatment for depression.[62] As such, it is suggested to be a viable treatment option. Since the meta-analysis by Zachariae and colleagues,[61] many trials have been published investigating an existing I-CBTI program (eg, Refs.[35–46,48,50–54,56,57,59,63–67]), and new programs have been introduced (eg, Refs.[45,47]). These studies reliably show positive effects (see **Table 3**).

The few direct comparisons that have been made between online and face-to-face CBTI have reported mixed results. Lancee and colleagues[52] found that face-to-face therapy substantially outperformed its online alternative. Blom and colleagues[36] compared I-CBTI with group therapy and did not report differences in effects. More research directly comparing face-to-face CBTI with I-CBTI is needed to compare effects of different treatment modalities and their moderators.

Effects of Internet-Delivered Cognitive Behavioral Therapy for Insomnia on Other (Mental) Health Symptoms and Daily Functioning

Insomnia is often comorbid with psychological complaints. Insomnia plays a role in the onset of anxiety disorders, bipolar disorders, and suicidality, but is most notably related to depression.[68] Patients suffering from a major depressive episode have an 80% chance of also reporting insomnia symptoms.[2] In addition, a person suffering from insomnia is at greater risk for depression.[69]

Table 3
Different Internet-delivered cognitive behavioral therapy for insomnia (all components) programs studied

Study	Program	Population	Scheduled Sessions	Support	Delivery	Indications of Effect Size[a]
Ström et al,[37] 2004	—	Adults	Order fixed, structured program at patients own[b] pace (5 sessions/wk)	Automated	Text-based	BAASS = 0.81.[37]
Suzuki et al,[35] 2008	—	Adults	Patients pick any 3 or more (4 sessions/2 wk)	Automated	Interactive Web platform	0.09–0.33 for SOL, TST, and SE.[35]
Vincent & Lewycky,[38] 2009	—	Adults	Fixed, structured program at patients own pace (5 sessions/6 wk)	None	Interactive Web platform	Range 0.14–0.75 for sleep diary variables.[38]
Espie et al,[39] 2012	Sleepio	Adults	Fixed, structured program at patients own pace (6 sessions/6 wk)	Automated, personalized	Interactive, virtual therapist	SCI = 0.89[50], SCI = 1.11.[51]
Lancee et al,[40] 2012	—	Adults	Fixed, structured program at patients own pace (6 sessions)	None	Text-based	ISI = 1.00[52], 1.05[43]; SLEEP50 Insomnia = 1.44[40]
Ho et al,[41] 2014	—	Adults	Fixed, structured program at patients own pace (6 sessions/6 wk)	Weekly phone support vs no support	Interactive Web platform	ISI = 0.53[41]
Van Straten et al,[42] 2014	I-Sleep	Adults	Fixed, structured program at patients own pace (text-based: 6[42], interactive: 5,[53] over 5–8 wk).	Weekly personal online therapist support	Text-based[42]; updated to interactive Web platform[53]	PSQI = 1.06[42]; ISI 2.36[53]

(continued on next page)

Table 3
(continued)

Study	Program	Population	Scheduled Sessions	Support	Delivery	Indications of Effect Size[a]
Blom et al,[36] 2015	—	Adults	Some elements fixed, some optional (8 sessions over 8 wk).	Weekly personal online therapist support	Text-based	ISI = 0.85[54], 1.8[36]
Thiart et al,[44] 2016	Get.On Recovery	Adults	Fixed, structured program at patients own pace (6 sessions)	Weekly personal online therapist support	Interactive Web platform	ISI = 1.45[55]
Bernstein et al,[45] 2017	GO! To sleep	Adults	Fixed, structured program at patients own pace (6 sessions/ 6 wk)	None	Interactive Web platform	n/a
Horsch et al,[47] 2017	Sleepcare	Adults	Fixed, structured program at patients own pace (6–7 wk)	Automated, personalized	Fully automated interactive app	ISI = 0.66[47]
Hagatun et al,[46] 2017; Ritterband et al,[48] 2017	SHUT-I	Adults	Fixed, structured program at patients own pace (6 sessions/ 6 wk)	Automated, personalized	Interactive Web platform	ISI = 1.14[56]
de Bruin et al,[49] 2015	—	Adolescents	Fixed weekly online sessions (6 sessions/6 wk)	Weekly personal feedback from a coach or therapist	Text-based	HSDQ insomnia scale = 1.26[49]

Abbreviations: BAASS, beliefs and attitudes about sleep scale; C-E, cost-effectiveness; ES, effect size; HSDQ, Holland sleep disorder questionnaire; ISI, insomnia severity index; n/a, not available; P HQ-9, patient health questionnaire-9; PSQI, Pittsburgh sleep quality index; SCI, sleep condition indicator; SE, sleep efficiency; SOL, sleep onset latency; TST, total sleep time; —, no specific title for this program.

[a] Between-group (cognitive behavioral therapy for insomnia vs placebo, wait list, or no treatment) Cohen's *d* reported from publications when available; reported effect sizes are between-group unless otherwise indicated; this is a selection of studies and not an exhaustive overview. For programs with more than 3 randomized controlled trials (RCTs) available, the effect sizes of the most recent 3 RCTs were reported. Reporting on insomnia severity measure when available; sleep diary otherwise; and different measure if neither are available.

[b] Patient-paced programs commonly have a 1 week per session minimum.

Residual insomnia complaints after successful depression treatment also predict depression relapse.[70]

Similar to face-to-face CBTI,[71,72] I-CBTI also has been shown to have antidepressant effects.[73] Most participants studied in these meta-analyses,[72,73] however, were not recruited for depression specifically, and severely depressed persons were not included in these studies. Three recent I-CBTI studies specifically assessing I-CBTI as a treatment for depressive symptoms and insomnia showed promising results. Blom and colleagues[57] found I-CBTI to be more effective than online depression treatment on insomnia and equally effective on depressive symptoms. Christensen and colleagues[64] and van der Zweerde and colleagues[53] demonstrated that I-CBTI reduced both depressive symptoms and insomnia symptoms in people suffering from both.[53,64]

Depressive symptoms are not the only psychiatric complaints influenced by I-CBTI. A large study by Freeman and colleagues[51] on 3755 students showed that I-CBTI also leads to positive changes in psychotic symptoms. Improving insomnia has been suggested to have beneficial effects on other aspects of (mental) health and quality of life as well.[50] This is particularly important because daytime complaints and impaired daily functioning are often the reason to seek treatment.[74] There is also evidence of I-CBTI improving work performance and cognitive complaints.[50,65,66]

FACTORS INFLUENCING INTERNET-DELIVERED COGNITIVE BEHAVIORAL THERAPY FOR INSOMNIA EFFECTS

Even though CBTI treatments are effective overall, the treatment does not work for everyone, up to an estimated 30% of persons with insomnia do not respond to treatment.[75] Why this is the case and which factors (eg, genetic, environmental, biological, lifestyle) play a role here is largely unknown. More research is needed to enable precision medicine approaches taking into account specific patient characteristics that influence the changes of treatment success.

Clear mediators and moderators of I-CBTI effects have yet to be determined. Some influential variables have been suggested by earlier research on CBTI (**Table 4**). It is yet unclear whether these factors differ between CBTI and I-CBTI, but it seems likely that comparable processes play a role in both treatment modalities.

Cognitive and Behavioral Factors

The importance of cognitive processes in insomnia treatment has been well documented

over the past 20 years (eg, Refs.[92–94]). Cognitive processes, such as worrying and dysfunctional beliefs, have been studied as mediators of the effects of CBTI treatment, with varying results.[43,56,76–80] Overall, although not all studies study the same specific outcomes and cognitive processes, cognitive factors do seem to play a role. Two important factors worth mentioning are insomnia-related worrying and dysfunctional beliefs.[81,95] Harvey[81] suggests patients with insomnia perceive worrying to be beneficial to them (which may in itself be seen as a dysfunctional belief). At the same time, worrying also heightens arousal, making sleeping difficult. Dysfunctional beliefs (eg, "Without a good night's rest I will not be able to function at work tomorrow") are a topic of worry, and can also aggravate the perceived consequences of poor sleep.

Behavioral factors such as habits incompatible with sleep, varying bedtimes, and spending too much time in bed are commonly seen among bad sleepers and influence effects of treatment. Harvey and colleagues[78] recently concluded that the effects of these behavioral factors depend on the type of treatment (behavioral treatment [BT], cognitive therapy [CT], or a combination) a person undergoes.[78] They observed that behavioral processes mediated the results for BT but not for CT. Notably, the cognitive mediators studied (worry, unhelpful beliefs about sleep, and monitoring behavior for sleep-related threat) were significant mediators of the effect of BT as well as CT. When patients report a high level of disturbance in both behavioral and cognitive sleep-related processes, they achieved better treatment results when they received the combined CBT.[78]

Delivery-Mode–Specific Factors

Online delivery may not be suited for everyone suffering from insomnia. Blom and colleagues[86] looked at patient-reported factors that facilitate and hinder uptake of I-CBTI. They found that having more than one psychological problem next to insomnia makes it more difficult to adhere to an I-CBTI program and may warrant different delivery modes or more intensive (human) support. A review on Internet therapy aimed at behavior changes emphasized that the intensity of a program should be high and that reminders, preferably text-messages, are important tools to enhance adherence.[88]

Sleep as a Perpetuating Factor in Other Psychiatric Problems

Disturbed sleep is seen in 60% of psychiatric patients,[96] and is often a perpetuating factor, for

Table 4
Factors that have been suggested to play a role in precision medicine for insomnia

Factors	Characteristic	Supported on Sequence	Level of Research Support
Mediators	Type of problem (cognitive or behavioral)	BT for primarily behavioral problems, CT for primarily cognitive problems, combined CBT when both are present.	• Empirical results on cognitive process vary,[43,56,76–80] their influence remains unclear. • Empirical evidence does show insomnia-related worrying and dysfunctional beliefs about sleep mediate treatment effects.[81] • Behavioral processes mediated results for BT, but not for CT in RCT.[78]
Predictors of treatment effects			
Demographic[a]	Age	Higher chance of treatment success with younger age.	• Meta-analytic evidence based on data from 49 studies.[82] • However: no evidence from older populations, age range in 90% of studies is quite small.[82]
	Educational level	Higher chance of treatment success with higher educational level.	• Observational study of intervention group only (Vincent et al, 2001) showed education moderated effects.[83] • Not found to moderate effects in meta-analysis.[82]
Clinical	Higher (>6 h) initial total sleep time[b]	Risk of dropout.	• Empirical evidence higher TST predicts dropout from dropped-out participants in RCT.[84]
	Lower initial total sleep time (<6 hr)	Lower chance of treatment success.	• Empirical evidence from RCT results.[85]
	Lower initial insomnia severity	Lower change of treatment success, may predict dropout.	• Empirical evidence from dropped-out participants in RCT.[84]
	Higher initial sleep efficiency[b]	Lower chance of treatment success.	• Suggested in 2014 conference abstract, results not published to our knowledge.[83]
	Other sleep disorders	Lower chance of treatment success.	• Observational study of intervention group only (Vincent et al, 2001) showed sleep comorbidity moderated effects.[83]
	Other psychiatric or medical disorders	Chance of lower adherence.	• Empirical RCT evidence shows psychiatric comorbidities warrant more intensive delivery modes/more intensive (human) support/scheduled program reminders. *(continued on next page)*

Factors	Characteristic	Supported on Sequence	Level of Research Support
			• Meta-analytic evidence of effect sizes equal to effect sizes in non-comorbid samples.[73] • Psychiatric comorbidities do not seem to decrease treatment effects and comorbidities may benefit from CBTI as well.[53,57,64,86–88] • Meta-analytic evidence shows the positive response to CBTI on insomnia symptoms does not appear to be moderated by the type of comorbid condition (psychiatric/medical).[89]
	Insomnia subtype	Different treatment (elements) may be indicated depending on for example, level of distress.	Insomnia subtypes identified by Blanken and colleagues,[90] further research and clinical application needed.

Table 4 (continued)

Abbreviations: BT, behavioral therapy; CBTI, cognitive behavioral therapy for insomnia; CT, cognitive therapy; RCT, randomized controlled trial; TST, total sleep time.

ᵃ Research suggests only 2.2% of variance in CBTI treatment effects on sleep efficiency (SE) was due to demographics (conference abstract by Espie and colleagues,[83] 2014).

ᵇ Paradoxical insomnia could also play a role when TST and/or SE are high but patients experience an insomnia problem nonetheless.[91]

example, in depression.[70] Treating insomnia also improves depression (eg, Refs.[53,64]); however, it is unclear how and why: more research into the mechanisms by which treating insomnia improves mood is needed. Often, mediation analysis is used to study such mechanisms (eg, Ref.[79]). To do this successfully, the mediator should be measured during and after intervention but before the effects occur and the sample size should be substantial.[97] I-CBTI has made it possible to do large trials adequately powered to assess mediation. These studies suggest that improvement of insomnia symptoms is preceding the improvements in depression (eg, Refs.[50,51]). Recently, network approaches have been developed to investigate changes in specific symptoms, instead of full questionnaires only. This new tool called Network Intervention Analysis (NIA[98]) can be used to study trial data using specific symptoms. This approach demonstrated that depression symptoms clear up *after* specific insomnia symptoms.[98] NIA could be used on other datasets in the field of I-CBTI to provide more insight into working mechanisms and hence into optimizing treatment response in patients with insomnia.

PERSONALIZING INTERNET-DELIVERED COGNITIVE BEHAVIORAL THERAPY FOR INSOMNIA

In psychotherapy, an important question is: what works for whom? As discussed previously, more knowledge on the working mechanisms of I-CBTI will likely lead to better treatments, but efficacy of the treatment also could depend on person-specific factors. It has been suggested that online CBT effects on anxiety and depression are moderated by age (older people reporting fewer beneficial effects) but not by other "person, problem, program, or provider characteristics."[82] For insomnia treatment, research by Cheng and colleagues[67] showed that I-CBTI effectively reduces symptoms across a wide range of demographic characteristics. Their large study was the first to identify different potential factors influencing the scope of treatment benefit, such as age, gender, socioeconomic status, and baseline severity, but also comorbidities in mental and physical health. They did not find any demographic variables to be associated with treatment efficacy and concluded that I-CBTI can be successfully offered to a wide and varied range of persons with insomnia complaints.[67] Luik and colleagues[83] suggested in their review that being younger and more highly educated improves one's chances of success.[99,100] They also reported on clinical predictors of treatment success. The limited available research suggests that comorbid sleep disorders other than insomnia, a higher initial sleep efficiency, lower baseline severity of insomnia, and longer total sleep time at the start of treatment may put a person at risk of improving little or not at all from I-CBTI.[83]

I-CBTI does not work for everyone suffering from insomnia.[75] The insomnia subtypes introduced by Blanken and colleagues[90] might offer a promising approach for tailoring treatment. Their 5 subtypes are as follows: (1) highly distressed; (2) moderately distressed, intact response to pleasurable emotions; (3) moderately distressed, weak response to pleasurable emotions; (4) low distress, low reactivity to environment and life events; and (5) low distress and high reactivity to environment and life events.[90] These stable subtypes have been shown to differ in biologically based traits and life history and treatment response.[90] Future research should focus on whether different insomnia treatments have different effects on the subtypes; that is, their clinical relevance. Specific subtypes may be present that will or will not respond well to I-CBTI. For example, a person whose subtype is particularly characterized by high presleep arousal might benefit more from mindfulness or acceptance-based techniques than from cognitive therapies.

COST-EFFECTIVENESS

Insomnia is a problem accompanied by substantial health care and societal costs, the latter for example, due to productivity loss and absence from work.[7] Treatment of insomnia could therefore potentially lead to large cost savings. Unfortunately, the cost-effectiveness of I-CBTI (or CBTI in general), has not been studied often. At least 3 studies have examined the cost-effectiveness of CBTI. These studies seem to suggest that the treatment is indeed cost-effective when offered in a face-to-face format,[101] to employees in online format,[44] and to adolescents online or in group format.[102] A pragmatic randomized controlled trial is currently under way studying whether I-CBTI can be offered cost-effectively in the general practice.[103]

IMPLEMENTATION

I-CBTI has several advantages that could facilitate implementation. It can be administered without scheduling appointments, and no travel time is required. This makes it suitable for those living remotely or with reduced mobility, limited time or busy schedules, and for those experiencing stigma preventing them from seeking face-to-face help. In addition, I-CBTI reduces waiting lists because much less resource is needed. However, online therapy also has some disadvantages that could impede implementation. A person has to invest a significant amount of time, which might require more self-discipline without face-to-face contact. In addition, people may have particular concerns about data privacy when data are shared online.[104] This makes it critical that programs adhere to respective regulations concerning data security. Also, not all persons suffering from insomnia may want online therapy: some insist on seeing a therapist, but equally some will prefer online treatment. Another concern might be related to personal safety. It may be preferable to keep a health care professional involved when a patient with insomnia is taking any online treatment. Automated systems can have algorithms to deal with certain safety issues. For example, when a program detects certain problems in the patient's answers (eg, suicide risk), patients could be automatically advised to contact their GP or health care professional, or a professional could be alerted to contact the patient automatically.

After determining effectiveness, working mechanisms, and costs associated with the treatment, the next big question is how best to implement online insomnia treatments. Whether or not a treatment is offered with or without support is an important factor in the implementation process. Accessible online treatments that are offered without human feedback are very scalable. Currently, a number of online programs can be freely purchased, but most programs are provided via research programs, health insurance programs, or at a (primary or secondary) care facility. Ideally, the guidelines recommending CBT for insomnia[31,32] should facilitate easy access to reimbursed treatment for diagnosed patients seeking help. Siversten and Nordgreen[105] have advised implementation of a varied range of modalities in which CBTI is offered, ranging from self-help material to online treatment to face-to-face conversations. Face-to-face therapy should then, due to scarcity of therapists, be provided only to those patients not helped (enough) through any of the other methods; that is, using a stepped-care approach.[105]

SUMMARY

There is ample evidence that I-CBTI is an effective treatment for those suffering from insomnia. This enables tailoring precision medicine to individual needs and characteristics. I-CBTI has the potential to play an important role in precision medicine because of its flexibility, accessibility, low costs, and multiple tailoring options. More research is needed looking into the moderators, mediators, and working mechanisms underlying the effects of I-CBTI on insomnia and other psychopathology to reach this potential. Then, we can offer efficacious treatment to those currently not benefiting from I-CBTI treatment, for reasons yet unknown. This would provide a strong incentive to implement I-CBTI on a larger scale, reaching more people, offering a true and perhaps preferable alternative to pharmacotherapy.

RESEARCH AGENDA

We suggest the following gaps in current research should be addressed:

1. Establishing patient characteristics influencing treatment success to facilitate a precision medicine approach.
2. Further specifying (sub)types of patients with insomnia and identifying optimal ways to offer subtype-specific treatment in a stepped-care and cost-effective manner.
3. Determining the working mechanisms of I-CBTI to be able to specifically target these in treatment.

REFERENCES

1. APA committee. Diagnostic and statistical manual of mental disorders, 5th edition: DSM-5. Washington, DC: American Psychiatric Association; 2013.
2. Ohayon MM. Epidemiology of insomnia: what we know and what we still need to learn. Sleep Med Rev 2002;6:97–111.
3. Morin CM, Bélanger L, LeBlanc M, et al. The natural history of insomnia: a population-based 3-year longitudinal study. Arch Intern Med 2009;169:447–53.
4. Baglioni C, Riemann D. Is chronic insomnia a precursor to major depression? Epidemiological and biological findings. Curr Psychiatry Rep 2012;14:511–8.
5. Suh S, Kim H, Yang HC, et al. Longitudinal course of depression scores with and without insomnia in non-depressed individuals: a 6-year follow-up longitudinal study in a Korean cohort. Sleep 2013;36:369–76.
6. Olfson M, Wall M, Liu SM, et al. Insomnia and impaired quality of life in the United States. J Clin Psychiatry 2018;79.
7. Daley M, Morin CM, LeBlanc M, et al. The economic burden of insomnia: direct and indirect costs for individuals with insomnia syndrome, insomnia symptoms, and good sleepers. Sleep 2009;32:55–64.
8. Kessler RC, Berglund PA, Coulouvrat C, et al. Insomnia and the performance of US workers: results from the America insomnia survey. Sleep 2011;34:1161–71.
9. Hoebert JM, Souverein PC, Mantel-Teeuwisse AK, et al. Reimbursement restriction and moderate decrease in benzodiazepine use in general practice. Ann Fam Med 2012;10:42–9.
10. Bertisch SM, Herzig SJ, Winkelman JW, et al. National use of prescription medications for insomnia: NHANES 1999-2010. Sleep 2014;37:343–9.
11. Glass J, Lanctôt KL, Herrmann N, et al. Sedative hypnotics in older people with insomnia: meta-analysis of risks and benefits. BMJ 2005;331:1169.
12. Buscemi N, Vandermeer B, Friesen C, et al. The efficacy and safety of drug treatments for chronic insomnia in adults: a meta-analysis of RCTs. J Gen Intern Med 2007;22:1335.
13. Manconi M, Ferri R, Miano S, et al. Sleep architecture in insomniacs with severe benzodiazepine abuse. Clin Neurophysiol 2017;128:875–81.
14. Hintze JP, Edinger JD. Hypnotic discontinuation in chronic insomnia. Sleep Med Clin 2018;13:263–70.
15. Holbrook AM, Crowther R, Lotter A, et al. Meta-analysis of benzodiazepine use in the treatment of insomnia. Can Med Assoc J 2000;162:225–33.
16. Smith MT, Perlis ML, Park A, et al. Comparative meta-analysis of pharmacotherapy and behavior therapy for persistent insomnia. Am J Psychiatry 2002;159:5–11.
17. Riemann D, Perlis ML. The treatments of chronic insomnia: a review of benzodiazepine receptor agonists and psychological and behavioral therapies. Sleep Med Clin 2009;13:205–14.
18. Everitt H, Baldwin D, Stuart B, et al. Antidepressants for insomnia in adults. New Jersey: Cochrane Library; 2018.
19. Kyle SD, Miller CB, Rogers Z, et al. Sleep restriction therapy for insomnia is associated with reduced objective total sleep time, increased daytime somnolence, and objectively impaired vigilance: implications for the clinical management of insomnia disorder. Sleep 2014;37:229–37.
20. American Academy of Sleep Medicine. International classification of sleep disorders. Diagnostic and coding manual 2005;2:51–5.
21. Morin CM, Espie CA. Insomnia: a clinical guide to assessment and treatment. New York: Springer Science & Business; 2007.
22. Murtagh DR, Greenwood KM. Identifying effective psychological treatments for insomnia: a meta-analysis. J Consult Clin Psychol 1995;63:79.
23. Edinger JD, Wohlgemuth WK. The significance and management of persistent primary insomnia: the

23. past, present and future of behavioral insomnia therapies. Sleep Med Rev 1999;3:101–8.

24. Harvey AG, Tang NK. Cognitive behaviour therapy for primary insomnia: can we rest yet? Sleep Med Rev 2003;7:237–62.

25. Montgomery P, Dennis J. A systematic review of non-pharmacological therapies for sleep problems in later life. Sleep Med Rev 2004;8:47–62.

26. Morin CM, Bootzin RR, Buysse DJ, et al. Psychological and behavioral treatment of insomnia: update of the recent evidence (1998–2004). Sleep 2006;29:1398–414.

27. Siebern AT, Suh S, Nowakowski S. Non-pharmacological treatment of insomnia. Neurotherapeutics 2012;9:717–27.

28. Trauer JM, Qian MY, Doyle JS, et al. Cognitive behavioral therapy for chronic insomnia: a systematic review and meta-analysis. Ann Intern Med 2015;163:191–204.

29. Van Straten A, van der Zweerde T, Kleiboer A, et al. Cognitive and behavioral therapies in the treatment of insomnia: a meta-analysis. Sleep Med Rev 2018; 38:3–16.

30. Van der Zweerde T, Bisdounis L, Kyle SD, et al. Cognitive behavioral therapy for insomnia: a meta-analysis of long-term effects in controlled studies. Under review.

31. Riemann D, Baglioni C, Bassetti C, et al. European guideline for the diagnosis and treatment of insomnia. J Sleep Res 2017;26:675–700.

32. Qaseem A, Kansagara D, Forciea MA, et al. Management of chronic insomnia disorder in adults: a clinical practice guideline from the American College of Physicians. Ann Intern Med 2016;165:125–33.

33. Morin CM, LeBlanc M, Daley M, et al. Epidemiology of insomnia: prevalence, self-help treatments, consultations, and determinants of help-seeking behaviors. Sleep Med 2006;7:123–30.

34. Everitt H, McDermott L, Leydon G, et al. GPs' management strategies for patients with insomnia: a survey and qualitative interview study. Br J Gen Pract 2014;64:112–9.

35. Suzuki E, Tsuchiya M, Hirokawa K, et al. Evaluation of an Internet-based self-help program for better quality of sleep among Japanese workers: a randomized controlled trial. J Occup Health 2008;50: 387–99.

36. Blom K, Tillgren HT, Wiklund T, et al. Internet- vs. group-delivered cognitive behavior therapy for insomnia: a randomized controlled non-inferiority trial. Behav Res Ther 2015;70:47–55.

37. Ström L, Pettersson R, Andersson G. Internet-based treatment for insomnia: a controlled evaluation. J Consult Clin Psychol 2004;72:113.

38. Vincent N, Lewycky S. Logging on for better sleep: RCT of the effectiveness of online treatment for insomnia. Sleep 2009;32:807–15.

39. Espie CA, Kyle SD, Williams C, et al. A randomized, placebo-controlled trial of online cognitive behavioral therapy for chronic insomnia disorder delivered via an automated media-rich web application. Sleep 2012;35:769–81.

40. Lancee J, van den Bout J, van Straten A, et al. Internet-delivered or mailed self-help treatment for insomnia? A randomized waiting-list controlled trial. Behav Res Ther 2012;50:22–9.

41. Ho FYY, Chung KF, Yeung WF, et al. Weekly brief phone support in self-help cognitive behavioral therapy for insomnia disorder: relevance to adherence and efficacy. Behav Res Ther 2014;63: 147–56.

42. Van Straten A, Emmelkamp J, De Wit J, et al. Guided Internet-delivered cognitive behavioural treatment for insomnia: a randomized trial. Psychol Med 2014;44:1521–32.

43. Lancee J, Eisma MC, van Straten A, et al. Sleep-related safety behaviors and dysfunctional beliefs mediate the efficacy of online CBT for insomnia: a randomized controlled trial. Cogn Behav Ther 2015;44:406–22.

44. Thiart H, Ebert DD, Lehr D, et al. Internet-based cognitive behavioral therapy for insomnia: a health economic evaluation. Sleep 2016;39: 1769.

45. Bernstein AM, Allexandre D, Bena J, et al. "Go! to sleep": a web-based therapy for insomnia. Telemed J E Health 2017;23:590–9.

46. Hagatun S, Vedaa Ø, Nordgreen T, et al. The short-term efficacy of an unguided Internet-based cognitive-behavioral therapy for insomnia: a randomized controlled trial with a six-month nonrandomized follow-up. Behav Sleep Med 2019;17(2):137–55.

47. Horsch CH, Lancee J, Griffioen-Both F, et al. Mobile phone-delivered cognitive behavioral therapy for insomnia: a randomized waitlist controlled trial. J Med Internet Res 2017;9. https://doi.org/10. 2196/jmir.6524.

48. Ritterband LM, Thorndike FP, Ingersoll KS, et al. Effect of a web-based cognitive behavior therapy for insomnia intervention with 1-year follow-up: a randomized clinical trial. JAMA Psychiatry 2017;74: 68–75.

49. de Bruin EJ, Bögels SM, Oort FJ, et al. Efficacy of cognitive behavioral therapy for insomnia in adolescents: a randomized controlled trial with Internet therapy, group therapy and a waiting list condition. Sleep 2015;38:1913–26.

50. Espie CA, Emsley R, Kyle SD, et al. Effect of digital cognitive behavioral therapy for insomnia on health, psychological well-being, and sleep-related quality of life: a randomized clinical trial. JAMA Psychiatry 2018. https://doi.org/10.1001/jamapsychiatry.2018.2745.

51. Freeman D, Sheaves B, Goodwin GM, et al. The effects of improving sleep on mental health (OASIS): a randomised controlled trial with mediation analysis. Lancet Psychiatry 2017;4:749–58.

52. Lancee J, van Straten A, Morina N, et al. Guided online or face-to-face cognitive behavioral treatment for insomnia: a randomized wait-list controlled trial. Sleep 2016;39:183–91.

53. Van der Zweerde T, Van Straten A, Effting M, et al. Does online insomnia treatment reduce depressive symptoms? A randomized controlled trial in individuals with both insomnia and depressive symptoms. Psychol Med 2019;49(3):501–9.

54. Kaldo V, Jernelöv S, Blom K, et al. Guided Internet cognitive behavioral therapy for insomnia compared to a control treatment–a randomized trial. Behav Res Ther 2015;71:90–100.

55. Thiart H, Lehr D, Ebert DD, et al. Log in and breathe out: Internet-based recovery training for sleepless employees with work-related strain–results of a randomized controlled trial. Scand J Work Environ Health 2015;41:164–74.

56. Chow PI, Ingersoll KS, Thorndike FP, et al. Cognitive mechanisms of sleep outcomes in a randomized clinical trial of Internet-based cognitive behavioral therapy for insomnia. Sleep Med 2018; 47:77–85.

57. Blom K, Jernelöv S, Kraepelien M, et al. Internet treatment addressing either insomnia or depression, for patients with both diagnoses: a randomized trial. Sleep 2015;38:267–77.

58. Spek V, Cuijpers PI, Nyklíček I, et al. Internet-based cognitive behaviour therapy for symptoms of depression and anxiety: a meta-analysis. Psychol Med 2007;33:319–28.

59. Lancee J, van den Bout J, Sorbi MJ, et al. Motivational support provided via email improves the effectiveness of Internet-delivered self-help treatment for insomnia: a randomized trial. Behav Res Ther 2013;51:797–805.

60. Jernelöv S, Lekander M, Blom K, et al. Efficacy of a behavioral self-help treatment with or without therapist guidance for co-morbid and primary insomnia—a randomized controlled trial. BMC Psychiatry 2012;12:5.

61. Zachariae R, Lyby MS, Ritterband LM, et al. Efficacy of Internet-delivered cognitive-behavioral therapy for insomnia–a systematic review and meta-analysis of randomized controlled trials. Sleep Med Rev 2016;30:1–10.

62. Andersson G, Cuijpers P. Internet-based and other computerized psychological treatments for adult depression: a meta-analysis. Cogn Behav Ther 2009;38:196–205.

63. Ritterband LM, Thorndike FP, Gonder-Frederick LA, et al. Efficacy of an Internet-based behavioral intervention for adults with insomnia. Arch Gen Psychiatry 2009;66:692–8.

64. Christensen H, Batterham PJ, Gosling JA, et al. Effectiveness of an online insomnia program (SHUTi) for prevention of depressive episodes (the GoodNight Study): a randomised controlled trial. Lancet Psychiatry 2016;3:333–41.

65. Bostock S, Luik AI, Espie CA. Sleep and productivity benefits of digital cognitive behavioral therapy for insomnia: a randomized controlled trial conducted in the workplace environment. J Occup Environ Med 2016;58:683–9.

66. Barnes CM, Miller JA, Bostock S. Helping employees sleep well: effects of cognitive behavioral therapy for insomnia on work outcomes. J Appl Psychol 2017;102:104.

67. Cheng P, Luik AI, Fellman-Couture C, et al. Efficacy of digital CBT for insomnia to reduce depression across demographic groups: a randomized trial. Psychol Med 2019;49:491–500.

68. Pigeon WR, Bishop TM, Krueger KM. Insomnia as a precipitating factor in new onset mental illness: a systematic review of recent findings. Curr Psychiatry Rep 2017;19:44.

69. Li MJ, Kechter A, Olmstead RE, et al. Sleep and mood in older adults: coinciding changes in insomnia and depression symptoms. Int Psychogeriatr 2018;30:431–5.

70. Carney CE, Segal ZV, Edinger JD, et al. A comparison of rates of residual insomnia symptoms following pharmacotherapy or cognitive-behavioral therapy for major depressive disorder. J Clin Psychiatry 2007;68:254–60.

71. Ballesio A, Aquino MRJV, Feige B, et al. The effectiveness of behavioural and cognitive behavioural therapies for insomnia on depressive and fatigue symptoms: a systematic review and network meta-analysis. Sleep Med Rev 2017;37: 114–29.

72. Gebara MA, Siripong N, DiNapoli EA, et al. Effect of insomnia treatments on depression: a systematic review and meta-analysis. Depress Anxiety 2018;35: 717–31.

73. Ye YY, Zhang YF, Chen J, et al. Internet-based cognitive behavioral therapy for insomnia (ICBT-i) improves comorbid anxiety and depression—a meta-analysis of randomized controlled trials. PLoS One 2015;10:e0142258.

74. Kyle SD, Crawford MR, Morgan K, et al. The Glasgow Sleep Impact Index (GSII): a novel patient-centered measure for assessing sleep-related quality of life impairment in insomnia disorder. Sleep Med 2013;14:493–501.

75. Morin CM, Benca R. Chronic insomnia. Lancet 2012;379:1129–41.

76. Okajima I, Nakajima S, Ochi M, et al. Reducing dysfunctional beliefs about sleep does not significantly improve insomnia in cognitive behavioral therapy. PLoS One 2014;9:e102565.

77. Espie CA, Kyle SD, Miller CB, et al. Attribution, cognition and psychopathology in persistent insomnia disorder: outcome and mediation analysis from a randomized placebo-controlled trial of online cognitive behavioural therapy. Sleep Med 2014;15:913–7.

78. Harvey AG, Dong L, Bélanger L, et al. Mediators and treatment matching in behavior therapy, cognitive therapy and cognitive behavior therapy for chronic insomnia. J Consult Clin Psychol 2017; 85:975.

79. Norell-Clarke A, Tillfors M, Jansson-Fröjmark M, et al. How does cognitive behavioral therapy for insomnia work? An investigation of cognitive processes and time in bed as outcomes and mediators in a sample with insomnia and depressive symptomatology. Int J Cogn Ther 2017;10:304–29.

80. Lancee J, Effting M, Van der Zweerde T, et al. Cognitive processes mediate the effects of insomnia treatment: evidence from a randomized wait-list controlled trial. Sleep Med 2019;54:86–93.

81. Harvey AG. A cognitive model of insomnia. Behav Res Ther 2002;40:869–93.

82. Grist R, Cavanagh K. Computerised cognitive behavioural therapy for common mental health disorders, what works, for whom under what circumstances? A systematic review and meta-analysis. J Contemp Psychother 2013;43: 243–51.

83. Espie CA, Bostock S, Kyle SD, et al. Who benefits from online CBT for insomnia? Factors associated with change in sleep efficiency in a large online treatment cohort. Sleep 2014;37:A205.

84. Yeung WF, Chung KF, Ho FYY, et al. Predictors of dropout from Internet-based self-help cognitive behavioral therapy for insomnia. Behav Res Ther 2015;73:19–24.

85. Bathgate CJ, Edinger J, Krystal AD. Insomnia patients with objective short sleep duration have a blunted response to cognitive behavioral therapy for insomnia. Sleep 2017;40.

86. Blom K, Jernelöv S, Lindefors N, et al. Facilitating and hindering factors in Internet-delivered treatment for insomnia and depression. Internet Interv 2016;4:51–60.

87. Dong L, Soehner AM, Bélanger L, et al. Treatment agreement, adherence, and outcome in cognitive behavioral treatments for insomnia. J Consult Clin Psychol 2018;86:294.

88. Webb TL, Joseph J, Yardley L, et al. Using the Internet to promote health behavior change: a systematic review and meta-analysis of the impact of theoretical basis, use of behavior change techniques, and mode of delivery on efficacy. J Med Internet Res 2010;12.

89. Wu JQ, Appleman ER, Salazar RD, et al. Cognitive behavioral therapy for insomnia comorbid with psychiatric and medical conditions: a meta-analysis. JAMA Intern Med 2015;175:1461–72.

90. Blanken TF, Benjamins JS, Borsboom D, et al. Robust insomnia disorder subtypes revealed by non-sleep-related traits and life history. Lancet Psychiatry 2019;6(2):151–63.

91. Castelnovo A, Ferri R, Punjabi NM, et al. The paradox of paradoxical insomnia: a theoretical review towards a unifying evidence-based definition. Sleep Med Rev 2018;44:70–82.

92. Perlis ML, Giles DE, Mendelson WB, et al. Psychophysiological insomnia: the behavioural model and a neurocognitive perspective. J Sleep Res 1997;6: 179–88.

93. Riemann D, Spiegelhalder K, Feige B, et al. The hyperarousal model of insomnia: a review of the concept and its evidence. Sleep Med Rev 2010;14:19–31.

94. Schwartz DR, Carney CE. Mediators of cognitive behavioral therapy for insomnia: a review of randomized controlled trials and secondary analysis studies. Clin Psychol Rev 2012;32:664–75.

95. Sunnhed R, Jansson-Fröjmark M. Are changes in worry associated with treatment response in cognitive behavioral therapy for insomnia? Cogn Behav Ther 2014;43:1–11.

96. Okuji Y, Matsuura M, Kawasaki N, et al. Prevalence of insomnia in various psychiatric diagnostic categories. Psychiatry Clin Neurosci 2002;56:239–40.

97. Kazdin AE. Understanding how and why psychotherapy leads to change. Psychother Res 2009; 19:418–28.

98. Blanken TF, Van der Zweerde T, Van Straten A, et al. Introducing Network Intervention Analysis to investigate sequential, symptom-specific treatment effects: a demonstration in co-occurring insomnia and depression. Psychother Psychosom 2019; 88(1):52–4.

99. Vincent N, Walsh K, Lewycky S. Determinants of success for computerized cognitive behavior therapy: examination of an insomnia program. Behav Sleep Med 2013;11:328–42.

100. Espie CA, Bostock S, Kyle SD, et al. Who benefits from online CBT for insomnia? Factors associated with change in sleep efficiency in a large online treatment cohort. Sleep 2014;37:A205.

101. Watanabe N, Furukawa TA, Shimodera S, et al. Cost-effectiveness of cognitive behavioral therapy for insomnia comorbid with depression: analysis of a randomized controlled trial. Psychiatry Clin Neurosci 2015;69:335–43.

102. De Bruin EJ, van Steensel FJ, Meijer AM. Cost effectiveness of group and Internet cognitive behavioral therapy for insomnia in adolescents: results from a randomized controlled trial. Sleep 2016;39:1571–81.

103. Van der Zweerde T, Lancee J, Slottje P, et al. Cost effectiveness of i-Sleep, a guided online CBT

intervention, for patients with insomnia in general practice: protocol of a pragmatic randomized controlled trial. BMC Psychiatry 2016;85.

104. Coulson NS, Smedley R, Bostock S, et al. The pros and cons of getting engaged in an online social community embedded within digital cognitive

behavioral therapy for insomnia: survey among users. J Med Internet Res 2016;18. https://doi.org/10.2196/jmir.5654.

105. Siversten B, Vedaa Ø, Nordgreen T. The future of insomnia treatment—the challenge of implementation. Sleep 2013;36:303–4.

Sleep Pharmacogenetics
The Promise of Precision Medicine

Andrew D. Krystal, MD, MS[a,b,]*, Aric A. Prather, PhD[a,1]

KEYWORDS

- Pharmacogenetics • Genetic polymorphism • Sleep disorder

KEY POINTS

- Pharmacogenetics is the branch of personalized medicine concerned with the variability in drug response occurring because of heredity.
- In recent years, advances in genetics research, including the mapping of the human genome and the increasing availability and decreasing costs of gene sequencing, have promoted tremendous growth in pharmacogenetics.
- There are several studies indicating that there are genetic influences on the outcomes of pharmacologic treatment of sleep disorders that seem ripe for application to clinical practice.
- Clinical implementation faces several challenges, including small effect sizes, perceived lack of clinical utility, the absence of effective guidelines for clinical application, and limited insurance reimbursement.
- The increasing availability and continued decreasing costs of genome sequencing and rapid development of research methods designed to improve the capacity to predict drug response fuel optimism that the existing limitations will be overcome and lead to an increasing capacity to apply pharmacogenetics to improve the treatment of individuals with sleep disorders.

INTRODUCTION

The concept of personalized or precision medicine is based on the observation that there is great variation among individuals in their clinical presentation, course of illness, and response to treatment.[1] Pharmacogenetics is the branch of personalized medicine concerned with the variability in drug response occurring because of heredity.[2] Pharmacogenetics goes back at least to Pythagoras who, in 510 BC, is credited with the observation that only some individuals died when eating fava beans.[3] The modern era of pharmacogenetics is reported to have begun in 1959 when an article was published using this term, which reported that drug-induced porphyria occurred only in a small subset of the population and that phenylthiourea is tasteless to some individuals and perceived as extremely bitter by others.[4] The aim of pharmacogenetics is to identify genetic variations that affect the response to pharmacotherapies so as to improve the capacity to predict who will have a favorable therapeutic response and who is predisposed to having adverse effects so that treatment can be tailored to each patient as a means of optimizing outcomes. Such genetic variations (**Table 1**) include (1) single nucleotide polymorphisms (SNPs), in which individuals vary in a single nucleotide at a specific position in the genome; (2) variable number tandem repeat

Disclosure: A. Krystal has received grants/research support from NIH, Janssen, Jazz, Axsome, Reveal Biosensors, and is a consultant for Adare, Eisai, Ferring, Galderma, Harmony Biosciences, Idorsia, Jazz, Janssen, Takeda, Merck, Neurocrine, Pernix, Physician's Seal. A. Prather has received grants/research support from NIH, Headspace Inc.
[a] University of California San Francisco, San Francisco, CA, USA; [b] Duke University School of Medicine, Durham, NC, USA
[1] Present address: 3333 California Street, San Francisco CA 94118.
* Corresponding author. 401 Parnassus Avenue, San Francisco, CA 94143.
E-mail address: andrew.krystal@ucsf.edu

Sleep Med Clin 14 (2019) 317–331
https://doi.org/10.1016/j.jsmc.2019.05.003
1556-407X/19/© 2019 Elsevier Inc. All rights reserved.

Table 1
Potential genetic variations

Genetic Variation	Definition
SNPs	Variation in a single nucleotide at a specific position in the genome
VNTR polymorphisms	Variation in the number of times a short sequence of nucleotides is repeated at a specific location in the genome
Copy number variants	Specific sections of the genome are repeated a variable number of times
Deletions	A sequence of DNA is absent from the genome
Insertions	One or more nucleotide base pairs is added into the genome

Abbreviations: SNPs, single nucleotide polymorphisms; VNTR, variable number tandem repeat.

(VNTR) polymorphisms, in which individuals vary in the number of times a short sequence of nucleotides is repeated at a specific location in the genome; (3) copy number variants, in which specific sections of the genome are repeated a variable number of times in individuals; (4) deletions, in which a sequence of DNA is lost during replication and absent from the genome, and; (5) insertions, in which 1 or more nucleotide base pairs is added into the DNA sequence.[5–8] These variations can affect drug response in a variety of ways, including by altering the function of drug receptors; ion channels affected by drug binding; a variety of enzymes, including enzymes that metabolize drugs; immune molecules; drug transporters; plasma protein binding of drugs; or proteins that synthesize, clear, or degrade the neurotransmitters that bind to the receptors that drugs bind to.[5]

In recent years, advances in genetics research, including the mapping of the human genome and the increasing availability and decreasing costs of gene sequencing, have promoted tremendous growth in pharmacogenetics. This growth has affected all areas of medicine, including sleep medicine, in which a growing body of research points to genetic factors that modulate the therapeutic and adverse responses to pharmacotherapy. This article reviews this body of work. It begins by providing a brief overview of sleep disorders and then identifies sleep disorders for which studies have been performed that have reported genetic variations that affect the therapeutic actions of agents or for which there is reason to believe that such an effect is likely and may have implications for a personalized medicine approach in caring for patients with sleep disorders.

OVERVIEW OF THE MAJOR SLEEP DISORDERS AND THEIR PRIMARY PHARMACOTHERAPIES

The Third Edition of the International Classification of Sleep Disorders (ICSD-3) identified 7 major categories of sleep disorders: insomnia, sleep-related breathing disorders, central disorders of hypersomnolence, circadian rhythm sleep-wake disorders, parasomnias, sleep-related movement disorders, and other sleep disorders.[9] With the exception of sleep-related breathing disorders, existing literature suggests that there are genetic variants that affect or are likely to affect the response to treatments for these sleep disorders. A brief overview of these sleep disorders are provided here.

Insomnia

The ICSD-3 defines 1 overarching condition, chronic insomnia disorder, which is defined as a report of persistent (at least 3 times per week for at least 3 months) difficulty falling or staying asleep in the context of the affected individual having an adequate opportunity and circumstances for sleep and associated daytime consequences.[9] There are a variety of pharmacologic treatments that are used to treat chronic insomnia disorder (**Table 2**).[10–1] These treatments include benzodiazepines, mechanistically related agents referred to as nonbenzodiazepines, selective histamine H1 receptor antagonists, hypocretin/orexin receptor antagonists, melatonin receptor agonists, nonselective histamine H1 receptor antagonists, antidepressants, antipsychotics, and anticonvulsants.

Benzodiazepines

The benzodiazepines are a group of chemically related compounds that are positive allosteric

Table 2
Medications used to treat sleep disorders

Medication Type	Mechanism of Action	Agents Most Commonly Used
Insomnia		
Benzodiazepines	GABA-A receptor positive allosteric modulation	Triazolam, temazepam, flurazepam, alprazolam, clonazepam, lorazepam
Nonbenzodiazepines	GABA-A receptor positive allosteric modulation	Zolpidem, zolpidem CR, transoral zolpidem, zaleplon, eszopiclone
Selective H1 antagonists	Antagonism of H1 histamine receptors	Doxepin 3–6 mg
Nonselective H1 antagonists	Antagonism of H1 histamine and acetylcholine receptors	Diphenhydramine, doxylamine
Hypocretin/orexin receptor antagonists	Antagonism of hypocretin/orexin receptors	Suvorexant
Melatonin receptor agonists	Agonists at MT1 and MT2 melatonin receptors	Ramelteon, melatonin
Antidepressants	Antagonism of serotonin transporter and a variety of other receptors	Trazodone, mirtazapine, amitriptyline, doxepin (in doses >6 mg), and trimipramine
Antipsychotics	Antagonism of dopamine D2 receptors and variety of other receptors	Quetiapine, olanzapine
N-type voltage-gated calcium channel modulators	Inhibiting N-type voltage-gated calcium channels by binding to alpha-2 subunit	Pregabalin, gabapentin
Central Disorders of Hypersomnolence		
Amphetamines	Stimulating release and inhibiting reuptake of norepinephrine and dopamine	Amphetamine/D-amphetamine and methamphetamine
Methylphenidate	Increases release of norepinephrine and dopamine	Methylphenidate
Modafinil	Mechanism of action thought to be inhibition of reuptake of norepinephrine and dopamine	Modafinil, R-modafinil
GABA-B agonists	Mechanism of wake promotion unknown	Sodium oxybate
Circadian Rhythm Sleep Disorders		
Melatonin receptor agonists	Agonists at MT1 and MT2 receptors, possibly intracellular melatonin receptors	Melatonin
Modafinil	Mechanism of action thought to be inhibition of reuptake of norepinephrine and dopamine	Modafinil, R-modafinil
Parasomnias		
Benzodiazepines	GABA-A receptor positive allosteric modulators	Clonazepam

(continued on next page)

Table 2
(continued)

Medication Type	Mechanism of Action	Agents Most Commonly Used
Sleep-related Movement Disorders		
Dopamine agonists	Agonists at dopamine D2, D3, and D4 receptors	Pramipexole, ropinirole
Dopamine precursors	Increase synthesis of dopamine	L-Dopa
N-type voltage-gated calcium channel modulators	Inhibiting N-type voltage-gated calcium channels by binding to alpha-2 subunit	Pregabalin, gabapentin

Abbreviations: CR, controlled release; GABA, gamma-aminobutyric acid.

modulators (PAMs) at the benzodiazepine binding site on the gamma-aminobutyric acid (GABA) type A receptor complex.[11–14] They exert a sleep-enhancing effect by potentiating GABA-A receptor–mediated inhibition. Benzodiazepines most commonly used to treat insomnia include triazolam, temazepam, flurazepam, alprazolam, clonazepam, and lorazepam.[14,15] Placebo-controlled trials indicate the efficacy of triazolam, temazepam, flurazepam, quazepam, and estazolam for sleep onset and maintenance difficulties.[14] These agents vary in their affinity to different types of GABA-A receptors in the brain.[16–18] As a result, they have differing clinical effects, which can include cognitive impairment, myorelaxant effects, antiseizure effects, and anxiolytic effects in addition to their sleep-enhancing effects.

Nonbenzodiazepines

Nonbenzodiazepines is a term used to refer to a group of medications that, like the benzodiazepines, are GABA-A receptor PAMs acting at the benzodiazepine binding site but are unrelated chemically to the benzodiazepines.[11–14] These agents include zolpidem, zolpidem CR (controlled release), zolpidem tartrate (sublingual), zaleplon, and eszopiclone. Their clinical effects are mediated by the same mechanism as the benzodiazepines and also vary in their clinical effects like the benzodiazepines because of variable binding to GABA-A receptors in the brain.[11–14,16–18] A sizable number of placebo-controlled trials have been performed that establish the efficacy and safety profiles of these agents in treating insomnia. Sleep onset effects have been documented for zolpidem and zaleplon, whereas sleep onset and maintenance therapeutic effects have been reported for zolpidem CR and eszopiclone.[14,19–24] Zolpidem tartrate and zaleplon have also been shown to have a favorable risk-benefit profile for middle-of-the-night administration.[25,26]

Selective histamine H1 receptor antagonists

The histamine H1 receptor exerts a wake-promoting effect when activated.[27] As a result, drugs that block this receptor can promote sleep.[27] Although many agents have H1 antagonist effects, nearly all of them do so nonselectively. The exceptions to this are doxepin in the 3-gm to 6-mg range of dosing and esmirtazapine (the S-isomer of mirtazapine) in a dose of 3 to 4.5 mg.[27–30] These two agents have H1 antagonism as by far their most potent effect. In higher doses used to treat depression (doxepin, ≥75 mg; mirtazapine, ≥15 mg) they have broad pharmacologic effects but, if the dose is low enough, they can have clinical effects only at the H1 receptor.[27] Studies with these medications in the range in which they have H1 selectivity show that H1 antagonism is associated with a unique set of effects, including greater effects on sleep maintenance than sleep onset, greatest effect size at the end of the night despite peak blood level occurring in the middle of the night, and a shortening of the time it takes to return to sleep without decreasing number of awakenings.[28–30]

Nonselective H1 antagonists

Several medications, are referred to as antihistamines, were developed to treat allergy problems but are frequently used to treat insomnia. As described earlier, these agents are not selective H1 antagonists in that they also block acetylcholine receptors with comparable potency as their H1 antagonist effects and this affects their sleep profile and also can lead to side effects.[27] Such agents include diphenhydramine and doxylamine, which are obtainable over the counter in the United States.[27] Double-blind placebo-controlled trials have only been performed with diphenhydramine and these are limited. These studies provide an indication that the effects may be more potent on maintenance than at onset.[27] One study of daytime dosing of diphenhydramine suggests that benefits versus placebo do not sustain beyond a few days; however, it remains unknown whether this is also true when diphenhydramine is taken at bedtime.[27]

Hypocretin/orexin receptor antagonists

Hypocretin/orexin receptor antagonists enhance sleep by blocking the wake-promoting effects of the peptide hypocretin/orexin.[31] One such agent, suvorexant, is U. Food and Drug Administration (FDA) approved for the treatment of insomnia and available in the United States. This agent has been shown to have robust efficacy and a favorable adverse effects profile in several double-blind, randomized, placebo-controlled studies.[31–36] The profile is somewhat reminiscent of doxepin in the 3-mg to 6-mg range in that the effects on sleep maintenance are more pronounced than on sleep onset onset effects of suvorexant are dose dependent), are greatest in the last third of the night, and decrease wake time without preventing awakenings.[31–36]

Melatonin receptor agonists

Melatonin is a hormone produced by the pineal gland that seems to have several physiologic effects, including that it seems to be related to circadian rhythmicity.[13] Melatonin agonists are thought to exert their therapeutic effects on sleep by binding to MT1 and MT2 melatonin receptors, which has been hypothesized to lead to a diminution of arousal systems emerging from the suprachiasmatic nucleus of the thalamus.[13,37] There are 2 melatonin agonists available for use in the United States: melatonin and ramelteon.[38] Melatonin is best established as a modulator of the circadian rhythm.[13] A large number of controlled studies have been performed on the effects of melatonin on insomnia symptoms in a variety of dosages and when given at various times with respect to sleep onset.[37,39,40] The studies do not generally provide robust evidence of a therapeutic effect on insomnia symptoms.[37,39–41] However, it does seem to have a consistent therapeutic effect in some populations, including those with neurodevelopmental disorders.[42–45] Ramelteon has been shown to have robust therapeutic effects in patients with insomnia but only for sleep onset problems, and the therapeutic effect is larger when measured with polysomnography than self-report assessment.[46] It does not seem to have abuse potential and has a favorable side effect profile.

Agents used off label to treat insomnia

A large number of agents of different types are not indicated for the treatment of insomnia but are used clinically for this purpose. These agents include antidepressants such as trazodone, mirtazapine, amitriptyline, doxepin (in doses >6 mg), and trimipramine; antipsychotics such as quetiapine and olanzapine; and anticonvulsants, including gabapentin and pregabalin.[12] The antidepressants and antipsychotics differ in their mechanisms of action but tend to have broad pharmacologic effects, including varying degrees of antagonism of histamine H1 receptors, α_1-adrenergic receptors, muscarinic cholinergic receptors, serotonin type 2 (5HT2) receptors, dopamine D2 receptors, and the serotonin transporter.[12] Gabapentin and pregabalin are thought to exert their primary effects by binding to the alpha-2-delta subunit of N-type voltage-gated calcium channels, thereby diminishing the level of activity of wake-promoting neurotransmitter systems, including glutamate and norepinephrine.[12] Although some of these agents are widely used to treat insomnia, most notably trazodone, the evidence base supporting their use in treating insomnia is limited. Double-blind placebo-controlled trials showing efficacy for the treatment of insomnia exist for the antidepressants trimipramine (50–200 mg; improved sleep quality and efficiency but not onset latency vs placebo) and doxepin (25–50 mg; improved sleep quality and onset and maintenance difficulties).[10,47–51]

Central Disorders of Hypersomnolence

This group of disorders consists of a set of conditions associated with excessive daytime sleepiness that is not caused by another sleep disorder, such as a breathing-related sleep disorder or a circadian rhythm disorder.[9] This group of disorders consists of narcolepsy, idiopathic hypersomnia, Kleine-Levin Syndrome, hypersomnia caused by a medical disorder, hypersomnia caused by a medication or substance, hypersomnia associated with a psychiatric disorder, and insufficient sleep syndrome.[9] Of these conditions, only 1 is associated with FDA-approved pharmacotherapies: narcolepsy. Although others of these conditions are sometimes treated with pharmacotherapy off label, those treatments are generally the same medications used to treat narcolepsy. As a result, this article discusses only treatments for narcolepsy, with the understanding that they are sometimes used to treat other hypersomnia disorders. In addition to excessive sleepiness, narcolepsy is also frequently associated with hypnogogic (occurring at sleep onset) or hypnopompic (occurring on waking) hallucinations and/or paralysis and cataplexy, a condition defined by episodes of sudden short-lived loss of muscle tone that are triggered by strong emotions, including fear, excitement, and laughter.[9]

Treatment of narcolepsy may include prescribing wake-promoting medications for the sleepiness and medications to target the other symptoms of narcolepsy.[52] Medications that are used to enhance wakefulness include amphetamine/D-amphetamine, methamphetamine, methylphenidate, modafinil, R-modafinil, and sodium oxybate. Amphetamine/D-amphetamine and methamphetamine are thought to enhance waking by stimulating release of norepinephrine and dopamine, and inhibiting the reuptake of these neurotransmitters.[52] Methylphenidate increases norepinephrine and dopamine release and has a lower risk of decreasing appetite and cardiovascular side effects than amphetamines but shares their abuse liability.[52] Although the mechanism of modafinil and R-modafinil are less well established, the available evidence suggests that they inhibit the reuptake of norepinephrine and serotonin.[52] Sodium oxybate is also used to treat sleepiness in patients with narcolepsy, although it works in a different way than the other wake-promoting medications. Its primary pharmacologic effect is binding to GABA-B receptors.[52] Notably, it is a sedating medication that is dosed at bedtime and has such a short half-life (0.5–1 hour) that it is redosed in the middle of the night. However, by unknown mechanism, it stimulates wakefulness the next day after nighttime dosing. It is hypothesized that this occurs via enhancing dopamine and norepinephrine release after it is eliminated.[52] This medication has also been shown to have a significant therapeutic effect on cataplexy during the day with nighttime dosing and is approved by the FDA for this purpose. Other medications used off label to treat cataplexy and other symptoms of narcolepsy other than sleepiness include antidepressants, including tricyclic antidepressants, selective serotonin reuptake inhibitors, and serotonin-norepinephrine reuptake inhibitors.[52]

Circadian Rhythm Sleep Disorders

This set of conditions includes delayed sleep-wake phase disorder, advanced sleep-wake phase disorder, irregular sleep-wake rhythm disorder, non–24-hour sleep-wake rhythm disorder, shift-work disorder, jet lag disorder, and circadian sleep-wake disorder not otherwise specified.[9] These disorders are defined as the presence of a least 3 months of difficulty (for all but jet lag disorder) consisting of a chronic or recurrent pattern of sleep-wake rhythm disruption primarily caused by an alteration in the endogenous circadian timing system or misalignment between the endogenous circadian rhythm and the sleep-wake schedule

desired or required, occurring in conjunction with insomnia or excessive sleepiness and associated with distress or impairment.[9] Treatments of these conditions include timed light exposure; timed melatonin administration; and, for shift-work sleep disorder, modafinil and R-modafinil.[53]

Parasomnias

Parasomnias consist of a group of recurrent episodic phenomena that occur during sleep. Some of these occur as partial arousals out of non–rapid eye movement (REM) sleep and are defined by incomplete awakening, alteration in responsiveness, diminished cognition (including no report of a dream experience), and some degree of amnesia for what occurred.[9] These include confusional arousals, sleepwalking, sleep terrors, and sleep-related eating disorder. Some individuals experience events during REM sleep, the most important of which are REM sleep behavior disorder, in which dream enactment occurs because of a loss of the usual paralysis that occurs during REM sleep, and nightmare disorder. The best-established and most commonly used treatment of both non-REM and REM parasomnias is the benzodiazepine clonazepam.[54]

Sleep-related Movement Disorders

The sleep-related movement disorders include stereotyped movements occurring during sleep as well as a dysesthesia that occurs during waking that prevents sleep from occurring (eg, restless legs syndrome).[9] The most important of these for the purposes of this article are restless legs syndrome (RLS), also known as Willis-Ekbom disease, and periodic limb movement disorder (PLMD). RLS is characterized by an urge to move the legs, sometimes accompanied by an uncomfortable sensation that occurs primarily with rest/inactivity and that is partially relieved by movement, for as long as the movement occurs; it occurs primarily in the evening or night and is associated with disturbance of sleep, distress, or daytime impairment.[55] PLMD is defined by repetitive dorsal flexion of the foot or flexion of the knee or hip occurring at least 15 times per hour in adults and associated with sleep disturbance or functional impairment.[9,55] Periodic limb movements occur in most patients with RLS. Therefore, it is not surprising that there is significant overlap in pharmacotherapy for these conditions. Dopamine agonists, including pramipexole, and ropinirole and the dopamine precursor L-dopa are considered first-line therapy for both conditions.[55,56] The alpha-2-delta calcium channel blockers gabapentin and pregabalin can also be used to treat these conditions and preliminary data support the use of clonazepam and melatonin for PLMD.[56]

GENETIC POLYMORPHISMS WITH POTENTIAL TO AFFECT ACTION OF TREATMENTS FOR SLEEP DISORDERS
Insomnia Therapies

There is some evidence that polymorphisms of liver cytochrome P450 (CYP) isoenzymes involved in the metabolism of some insomnia therapies affect optimal dosing in terms of achieving an optimal therapeutic effect and avoiding adverse effects, including daytime impairment (**Table 3**). Although some animal data indicate that there are genetic variations in GABA-A receptor constituent peptide among individuals that have been reported to affect the responsivity of mice to benzodiazepines and nonbenzodiazepines, there is no evidence that this is the case in humans.[57–59]

Zolpidem

Zolpidem is among the best examples of a drug with clinically important differences in subgroups of the population. Women have been noted to have a higher incidence of adverse effects with zolpidem than men, including greater morning sedation and higher rates of abuse, dependence, and withdrawal.[60–65] Further, women have been found to show greater impairment in automobile driving after receiving zolpidem during the day and in the morning after receiving zolpidem in the middle of the night.[63] Based on such observations, the FDA recommended halving the initial dose of zolpidem in all forms for women.[66]

The sex difference in zolpidem adverse effects is grounded in differences in pharmacokinetics. Zolpidem absorption seems to be greater in women and clearance is slower, such that women experience significantly higher blood levels (area under the curve is approximately 50% higher in women vs men receiving the same dose); an effect that is not explained by differences in body weight.[64,65,67,68]

There has been some debate about the mechanism responsible for the sex difference in zolpidem pharmacokinetics. The key steps in the metabolism of zolpidem are thought to be its hydroxylation by CYP3A4, its oxidation to an aldehyde by alcohol dehydrogenases (ADHs), and its conversion into a carboxylic acid by aldehyde dehydrogenases (ALDHs).[69,70] Some clinicians have argued for a role of sex differences in CYP3A4 activity; however, this is implausible because several drugs primarily metabolized by this liver enzyme do not manifest sex differences in pharmacokinetics and, if anything, CYP3A4 activity is greater

in women than in men.[71] Instead, the evidence suggests that lesser activity of ADHs and ALDHs in women is responsible for the greater absorption and slower elimination of zolpidem.[72] ADHs and ALDHs are well known to have double the activity in male versus female humans and rats.[73,74] More direct evidence for the role of ADHs and ALDHs is that the absorption and elimination of zolpidem in male rats became comparable with that in female rats following both castration and administration of a blocker of ADHs/ALDHs (Peer and colleagues,[72] 2016).

Clonazepam
Clonazepam is metabolized primarily by CYP3A4 into 7-amonoclonazepam, which undergoes a second stage of metabolism via acetylation by NAT2 (N-acetyl transferase 2).[75] There are polymorphisms in the population of NAT2 that lead to decreased efficacy of this acetylation and results in greater blood levels and, therefore, greater risks for side effects, such as daytime sedation/impairment for a given dose of clonazepam.[75]

Lorazepam
Similar to clonazepam, lorazepam undergoes a second stage of metabolism by UGT (UDP-glucuronosyltransferase). Polymorphisms of UGT genes in the population include some forms of UGT that are less effective in eliminating lorazepam, thereby increasing the likelihood of adverse effects in affected individuals, as documented in a recent case report.[76]

Diphenhydramine
Multiple CYP450 isoenzymes are involved in metabolizing diphenhydramine, including CPY2D6, CYP1A2, CYP2C9, and CYP2C19.[77] Polymorphisms of CYP2D6 have been reported to affect the clinical effects of this medication and are thought to be responsible, at least to a degree, for observed variability in clinical treatment outcomes.[5] Those with more effective CYP2D6 metabolize diphenhydramine very rapidly and have been reported to experience a countertherapeutic excitation when treated with this medication.[78] A CYP2D6 polymorphism that is associated with less effective metabolism (CYP2D6*10) is associated with an increased risk for daytime sleepiness.[5,79]

Doxepin
There are variants in the population in 2 of the main enzymes involved in the metabolism of doxepin, CYP2D6, CYP2D9, and CYP2C19, which lead to variability in both therapeutic and adverse effects among treated individuals.[5,80]

Table 3
Genetic polymorphisms with potential to affect action of treatments for sleep disorders

Medication	Polymorphism	Potential Clinical Effect
Insomnia		
Zolpidem	Not a polymorphism; sex hormone-related enhancement of activity of ADHs/ALDHs (involved in degradation of zolpidem) in men	Higher blood levels in women vs men at the same dose. Potential for increased side effects in women and lack of efficacy in men
Clonazepam	Loss-of-function polymorphism of NAT2 (N-acetyl transferase 2) involved in metabolism of clonazepam	Increases blood levels in affected individuals with potential for adverse effects
Lorazepam	Loss-of-function polymorphism of UGT involved in metabolism of lorazepam	Increases blood levels in affected individuals with potential for adverse effects
Diphenhydramine	Polymorphisms of CYP2D6 (involved in metabolism of diphenhydramine) exist that increase and decrease efficacy of metabolism	Affected individuals may have increased risk of side effects or loss of efficacy depending on type of polymorphism
Doxepin	Polymorphisms exist of 2 main enzymes in metabolism: CYP2D6 and CYP2D9, associated with increased and decreased efficacy of metabolism	Affected individuals may have increased risk of side effects or loss of efficacy depending on type of polymorphism
Trazodone	Polymorphisms exist in the 3 main enzymes involved in the degradation of this trazodone: CYP3A4, CYP2D6, and CYP1A2	Those with more effective CYP1A2 and CYP3A4 may experience inadequate therapeutic effects at a dosage at which benefit often occurs and those with less effective activity of these isoenzymes are likely to experience increased risk of adverse effects. Those with relatively effective CYP3A4 but relative inactivity of CYP2D6 experience buildup of mCPP and can experience stimulantlike effects, anxiety, shivering, dizziness, and heightened sensitivity toward light and noise
Central Disorders of Hypersomnolence		
Amphetamines, methylphenidate, modafinil	VNTR polymorphism exists in the SLC6A3 gene coding for the dopamine transporter, which affects clinical effects occurring with agents that block this transporter (amphetamines, modafinil); common SNP exists in the gene for an enzyme that breaks down dopamine (catechol O-methyl transferase COMT), which leads to variation in dopamine levels and cortical dopamine tone	Dopamine transporter polymorphisms associated with greater clinical effects in a subset of the population associated with greater risks of side effects such as psychosis COMT polymorphisms lead some individuals to experience lack of efficacy with these agents and others to be prone to adverse effects

(continued on next page)

Table 3
(continued)

Medication	Polymorphism	Potential Clinical Effect
Circadian Rhythm Sleep Disorders		
Melatonin	An SNP of a key enzyme involved in metabolism of melatonin (CYP1A2) leads some individuals to have significantly lower melatonin blood levels	Affected individuals have a lessened therapeutic response to melatonin
Parasomnias		
Clonazepam	Loss-of-function polymorphism of NAT2, involved in metabolism of clonazepam	Increases blood levels in affected individuals, with potential for adverse effects
Sleep-related Movement Disorders		
L-Dopa	SNPS affecting COMT activity exist; there are also variations in the gene for the MAO -B, which is also involved in breakdown of dopamine	Individuals with low COMT activity are at risk for L-dopa–induced dyskinesia; those with high COMT activity require higher doses to achieve a therapeutic effects Similar to COMT, those with low MAO-B activity are at risk for dyskinesia; Those with high MAO-B activity require higher doses to achieve a therapeutic effects
Dopamine agonists	Polymorphisms in CYP1A2, primary enzyme involved in ropinirole metabolism lead to variations in ropinirole blood levels Polymorphisms of the gene for SLC22A1 (involved in pramipexole metabolism) affect pramipexole blood levels DRD3 polymorphisms alter the effects of pramipexole	Those with more effective CYP1A2 are prone to adverse effects with ropinirole Those with more effective SLC22A1 require higher pramipexole dosage Individuals with particular DRD3 polymorphisms require a higher dosage of pramipexole

Abbreviations: ADH, alcohol dehydrogenase; ALDH, aldehyde dehydrogenase; COMT, catechol O-methyl transferase; DRD3, dopamine receptor type 3; MAO, monoamine oxidase; mCPP, methyl-chlorophenylpiperazine; NAT2, N-acetyl transferase 2; UGT, UDP-glucuronosyltransferase.

Trazodone

Trazodone has long been established to be associated with significant interindividual variation in metabolism, with a half-life ranging from 2.6 to 11 hours.[81–86] Key factors responsible for this are polymorphisms in the population of the enzymes involved in the degradation of this molecule: CYP3A4, CYP2D6, and CYP1A2.[81,82,85,86] Trazodone is cleaved into methyl-chlorophenylpiperazine (mCPP), an active metabolite, and an inactive metabolite by CYP3A4.[86] Trazodone is also metabolized by CYP1A2 into another inactive metabolite.[85] As a result, polymorphisms in either of these enzymes can affect blood levels of trazodone. Those with more effective CYP1A2 and CYP3A4 may experience inadequate therapeutic effects at a dosage at which benefit often occurs, and those with less effective activity of these isoenzymes are likely to experience increased risk of adverse effects.[87] Speaking to the clinical relevance of such effects, CYP3A4 levels vary 5-fold to 20-fold in the population.

The fact that trazodone has an active metabolite, mCPP, adds significant complexity to clinical management because mCPP has effects that are in some ways the opposite of what the patients are hoping to experience when taking trazodone for treating their insomnia. mCPP is a serotonergic postsynaptic receptor agonist (5-HT1 and 5-HT2) and is a drug of abuse that is closely related to ecstasy (methylenedioxymethamphetamine [MDMA]).[82,88,89] The effects of mCPP, which include stimulantlike effects, anxiety, shivering, dizziness, heightened sensitivity toward light and noise, are highly unexpected by patients with insomnia receiving this medication and can be extremely upsetting.[82,88,89]

Because CYP3A4 is responsible for the production of mCPP from trazodone, individuals with polymorphisms of this isoenzyme that are more effective are at increased risk for experiencing mCPP effects with treatment. This risk is particularly heightened in those with relatively effective CYP3A4 but relative inactivity of CYP2D6, the isoenzyme responsible for inactivating mCPP.[86] The available data suggest that 1% of the population are CYP2D6 ultrarapid metabolizers, 7% to 10% of white people are poor metabolizers, whereas Asians and Africans are less likely to have a low level of CYP2D6 activity.[90]

It should be clear from the considerations discussed earlier that the optimal use of trazodone involves a higher degree of complexity than most other medications. Achieving optimal clinical outcomes with trazodone requires starting with the lowest possible dose, titrating the dose slowly as needed, and warning patients of the possibility of mCPP-mediated effects, including activation and anxiety.

Hypocretin/orexin receptor antagonists

Genetic polymorphisms have been identified that affect the synthesis of hypocretin/orexin and hypocretin/orexin type 1 and 2 receptors.[91] However, it is currently unclear whether these variants affect the clinical effects of antagonists of hypocretin/orexin receptors used to treat insomnia.[5]

Therapies for Central Disorders of Hypersomnolence

Stimulants

Clinically relevant polymorphisms exist for 2 mechanisms related to the effects of stimulants: the dopamine (DAT) transporter, which is inhibited by some of these agents, and the enzyme catechol-O-methyltransferase (COMT), responsible for breaking down central dopamine, levels of which are increased by several stimulant agents.[5] The relevant DAT transporter polymorphisms have a VNTR in the SLC6A3 gene coding for the DAT; the most common and clinically important of these are 10-repeat (*10R) and 9-repeat (*9R) polymorphisms.[92] Observations of the clinical effects of these polymorphisms suggest greater clinical effects in the *9R compared

with *10R allele and include a greater likelihood of psychosis occurring with methamphetamine,[93] and a greater functional MRI neural response during a go-no-go task.[94]

The relevant COMT polymorphism is a common SNP occurring at codon 158 in the COMT gene.[95] The met allele of the val158met SNP, which causes a substitution of the amino acid methionine for valine, is associated with a significant reduction in COMT activity compared with the val allele and results in significantly increased cortical dopamine tone.[95] Observations of greater clinical effects of stimulants in val compared with met individuals include that modafinil given during sleep deprivation led to maintenance of baseline performance on several cognitive tests throughout sleep deprivation in val/val homozygotes, whereas minimal effects of modafinil were noted in met/met homozygotes[96]; and D-amphetamine was found to improve attention and processing speed performance in both val/val and val/met individuals, but not in met/met homozygotes.[97] An additional observation that seems to suggest that there is complexity to understanding the clinical effects of these alleles is that the treatment of daytime sleepiness in those with narcolepsy required a significantly greater daily dose of modafinil in val/val homozygotes compared with met/met individuals.[98]

Based on these observations, it should be expected that some individuals in the population will be prone to adverse effects with D-amphetamine such that lower dosages would be indicated, modafinil and D-amphetamine will fail to have therapeutic effects on sleepiness in some individuals, and modafinil doses in narcolepsy will need to be higher in some individuals than others.

Circadian Rhythm Disorders

Melatonin

Melatonin metabolism is primarily driven by CYP1A2.[99] An SNP of CYP1A2 has been found to affect CYP1A2 activity such that individuals who are homozygous for the *1A allele, which is associated with lesser CYP1A2 activity, have higher blood levels of melatonin than *1F homozygotes.[99] Clinically, *1F homozygotes have been reported to have fewer therapeutic sleep effects from melatonin than *1A homozygotes and heterozygotes.[100]

Parasomnias

Clonazepam

As described earlier related to insomnia, polymorphisms of NAT2, which is responsible for the second stage of metabolism of clonazepam, vary in their effectiveness such that the less effective polymorphism is associated with increased clonazepam blood levels and greater risks of adverse effects.[75]

Sleep-related Movement Disorders

L-Dopa

There is no direct evidence indicating whether genetic polymorphisms affect the clinical effects of L-dopa when used to treat sleep-related movement disorders. However, there is some evidence that there are polymorphisms affecting clinical effects when this agent is used to treat Parkinson disease (PD).[101–104] Given that L-dopa is broken down by COMT, it is not surprising that the effective dose of L-dopa when used to treat PD differs as a function of SNPs altering the effectiveness of this enzyme.[101,104] Patients with PD with SNPs associated with high COMT activity have been found to require higher doses of L-dopa to achieve therapeutic effects.[101,104] Genetic variations in COMT also affect the risk of L-dopa–induced dyskinesia. Individuals who are LL homozygotes for the COMT rs4680 gene were more likely to experience this adverse effect, whereas the C allele of the rs393795 gene was associated with a greater time until the onset of dyskinesia.[103] The activity of monoamine oxidase enzymes also affects the clinical effects of L-dopa. The basis for this is that the clinical effects of L-dopa are thought to be mediated by increasing dopamine synthesis and dopamine is degraded by monoamine oxidase enzymes. Greater doses of L-dopa seem to be required for the treatment of patients with PD who carry the monoamine oxidase (MAO)-B G allele and who have high MAO-A enzyme activity, and a greater risk of dyskinesia with L-dopa was reported for individuals with A and AA genotypes of the MAO-B rs1799836 gene.[103,104]

Dopamine agonists

There are no studies rigorously assessing whether polymorphisms of genes encoding for key enzymes degrading dopamine agonists have clinical effects. However, because the enzyme primarily involved in ropinirole metabolism is CYP1A2, which varies in effectiveness because of polymorphisms in the population, it seems likely that individuals with less effective CYP1A2 will be prone to adverse effects and be best treated with a lower dosage than those with more effective CP1A2.[5,105,106]

It has reported that there are clinical effects of polymorphisms of the SLC22A1 gene, which encodes for the organic cation transporter 1, for which pramipexole is a substrate.[107] The rs622342 A polymorphism is associated with higher prescribed dosages of pramipexole and possibly other medications used to treat PD than the C polymorphism.[107]

Polymorphisms of dopamine receptor genes have also been studied to determine whether they influence the clinical effects of dopamine agonists. Two studies suggested that dopamine receptor type 3 (DRD3) Ser9Gly polymorphisms influence the effects of pramipexole such that Gly/Gly homozygotes required higher pramipexole doses than Ser/Gly and Ser/Ser individuals.[108,109]

SUMMARY

The genetic influences on the treatment of sleep disorders described earlier seem ripe for application to clinical practice. However, clinical implementation faces several challenges in the clinical application of pharmacogenetic findings in all areas of medicine (Scott,[1] 2011). These challenges include small effect sizes, perceived lack of clinical utility, the absence of effective guidelines for clinical application, and limited insurance reimbursement (Scott,[1] 2011). Several trials have been performed and are in progress attempting to define/establish clinical utility, but these have so far had limited impact. However, the increasing availability and continued decreasing costs of genome sequencing and rapid development of research methods designed to improve the capacity to predict drug response fuel optimism that the existing limitations will be overcome and lead to an increasing capacity to apply pharmacogenetics to tailor the treatment of sleep disorders in individuals.

REFERENCES

1. Scott SA. Personalizing medicine with clinical pharmacogenetics. Genet Med 2011;13(12):987–95.
2. Pirmohamed M. Pharmacogenetics and pharmacogenomics. Br J Clin Pharmacol 2001;52:345–7.
3. Nebert DW. Pharmacogenetics and pharmacogenomics: why is this relevant to the clinical geneticist? Clin Genet 1999;56:247–58.
4. Vogel F. Moderne Probleme der Humangenetik. In: Heilmeyer L, Schoen R, de Rudder B, editors. Ergebnisse der Inneren Medizin und Kinderheilkunde. Ergebnisse der Inneren Medizin und Kinderheilkunde, vol 12. Heidelberg: Springer, Berlin; 1959.
5. Landolt HP, Holst SC, Valomon A. Clinical and experimental human sleep-wake pharmacogenetics. Handb Exp Pharmacol 2018. [Epub ahead of print].

6. Sadee W, Dai Z. Pharmacogenetics/genomics and personalized medicine. Hum Mol Genet 2005;14: R207–14.

7. Roden DM, Wilke RA, Kroemer HK, et al. Pharmacogenomics the genetics of variable drug responses. Circulation 2011;123:1661–70.

8. Holst SC, Valomon A, Landolt HP. Sleep pharmacogenetics: personalized sleep-wake therapy. Annu Rev Pharmacol Toxicol 2016;56:577–603.

9. American Academy of Sleep Medicine. International classification of sleep disorders. 3rd edition. Darien (IL): American Academy of Sleep Medicine; 2014.

10. Sateia MJ, Buysse DJ, Krystal AD, et al. Clinical practice guideline for the pharmacologic treatment of chronic insomnia in adults: an American Academy of Sleep Medicine Clinical Practice Guideline. J Clin Sleep Med 2017;13(2):307–49.

11. Krystal AD. Current, emerging, and newly available insomnia medications. J Clin Psychiatry 2015; 76(8):e1045.

12. Minkel J, Krystal AD. Optimizing the pharmacologic treatment of insomnia: current status and future horizons. Sleep Med Clin 2013;8(3):333–50.

13. Richey SM, Krystal AD. Pharmacological advances in the treatment of insomnia. Curr Pharm Des 2011; 17(15):1471–5.

14. Krystal AD. A compendium of placebo-controlled trials of the risks/benefits of pharmacological treatments for insomnia: the empirical basis for US clinical practice. Sleep Med Rev 2009;13(4):265–74.

15. Walsh JK. Drugs used to treat insomnia in 2002: regulatory-based rather than evidence-based medicine. Sleep 2004;27(8):14441–2.

16. Sieghart W, Sperk G. Subunit composition, distribution and function of GABA(A) receptor subtypes. Curr Top Med Chem 2002;2:795–816.

17. Sanna E, Busonero F, Talani G, et al. Comparison of the effects of zaleplon, zolpidem, and triazolam at various GABA(A) receptor subtypes. Eur J Pharmacol 2002;451(2):103–10.

18. Jia F, Goldstein PA, Harrison NL. The modulation of synaptic GABA(A) receptors in the thalamus by eszopiclone and zolpidem. J Pharmacol Exp Ther 2009;328(3):1000–6.

19. Krystal AD, Walsh JK, Laska E, et al. Sustained efficacy of eszopiclone over six months of nightly treatment: results of a randomized, double-blind, placebo controlled study in adults with chronic insomnia. Sleep 2003;26:793–9.

20. Walsh J, Krystal AD, Amato DA. Nightly treatment of primary insomnia with eszopiclone for six months: effect on sleep, quality of life and work limitations. Sleep 2007;30(8):959–68.

21. Krystal AD, Erman M, Zammit GK, et al. Long-term efficacy and safety of zolpidem extended-release 12.5 mg, administered 3 to 7 nights per week for 24 weeks, in patients with chronic primary insomnia: a 6-month, randomized, double-blind, placebo-controlled, parallel-group, multicenter study. Sleep 2008;31(1):79–90.

22. Fava M, McCall WV, Krystal A, et al. Eszopiclone Co-administered with fluoxetine in patents with insomnia Co-existing with major depressive disorder. Biol Psychiatry 2006;59:1052–60.

23. Pollack M, Kinrys G, Krystal A, et al. Eszopiclone co-administered with escitalopram in patients with insomnia and comorbid generalized anxiety disorder. Arch Gen Psychiatry 2008;65(5):551–62.

24. Goforth HW, Preud'homme XA, Krystal AD. A randomized, double-blind, placebo-controlled trial of eszopiclone for the treatment of insomnia in patients with chronic low back pain. Sleep 2014;37(6):1053–60.

25. Roth T, Krystal A, Steinberg FJ, et al. Novel sublingual low-dose zolpidem tablet reduces latency to sleep onset following spontaneous middle-of-the-night awakening in insomnia in a randomized, double-blind, placebo-controlled, outpatient study. Sleep 2013;36(2):189–96.

26. Zammit GK, Corser B, Doghramji K, et al. Sleep and residual sedation after administration of zaleplon, zolpidem, and placebo during experimental middle-of-the-night awakening. J Clin Sleep Med 2006;2(4):417–23.

27. Krystal AD, Richelson E, Roth T. Review of the histamine system and the clinical effects of H1 antagonists: basis for a new model for understanding the effects of insomnia medications. Sleep Med Rev 2013;17(4):263–72.

28. Krystal AD, Durrence HH, Scharf M, et al. Efficacy and safety of doxepin 1 mg and 3 mg in a 12-week sleep laboratory and outpatient trial of elderly subjects with chronic primary insomnia. Sleep 2010; 33(11):1553–61.

29. Krystal AD, Lankford A, Durrence HH, et al. Efficacy and safety of doxepin 3 and 6 mg in a 35-day sleep laboratory trial in adults with chronic primary insomnia. Sleep 2011;34(10):1433.

30. Ivgy-May N, Ruwe F, Krystal A, et al. Esmirtazapine in non-elderly adult patients with primary insomnia: efficacy and safety from a randomized, 6-week sleep laboratory trial. Sleep Med 2015;16(7): 838–44.

31. Herring WJ, Connor KM, Ivgy-May N, et al. Suvorexant in patients with insomnia: results from two 3-month randomized controlled clinical trials. Biol Psychiatry 2016;79(2):136–48.

32. Michelson D, Snyder E, Paradis E, et al. Safety and efficacy of suvorexant during 1-year treatment of insomnia with subsequent abrupt treatment discontinuation: a phase 3 randomised, double-blind, placebo-controlled trial. Lancet Neurol 2014;13(5):461–71.

33. Herring WJ, Connor KM, Snyder E, et al. Suvorexant in patients with insomnia: pooled analyses of three-month data from phase-3 randomized controlled clinical trials. J Clin Sleep Med 2016; 12(9):1215–25.

34. Herring WJ, Connor KM, Snyder E, et al. Clinical profile of suvorexant for the treatment of insomnia over 3 months in women and men: subgroup analysis of pooled phase-3 data. Psychopharmacology (Berl) 2017;234(11):1703–11.

35. Herring WJ, Connor KM, Snyder E, et al. Suvorexant in elderly patients with insomnia: pooled analyses of data from phase III randomized controlled clinical trials. Am J Geriatr Psychiatry 2017;25(7):791–802.

36. Herring WJ, Roth T, Krystal AD, et al. Orexin receptor antagonists for the treatment of insomnia and potential treatment of other neuropsychiatric indications. J Sleep Res 2018;28:e12782.

37. Sack R, Hughes RJ, Edgar DM, et al. Sleep-promoting effects of melatonin: at what dose, in whom, under what conditions, and by what mechanisms? Sleep 1997;20(10):908–15.

38. Morin CM, Drake C, Harvey AG, et al. Insomnia disorder. Nat Rev Dis Primers 2015;1:15026.

39. Ferracioli-Oda E, Qawasmi A, Bloch MH. Meta-analysis: melatonin for the treatment of primary sleep disorders. PLoS One 2013;8:e63773.

40. Buscemi N, Vandermeer B, Hooton N, et al. The efficacy and safety of exogenous melatonin for primary sleep disorders. A meta-analysis. J Gen Intern Med 2005;20(12):1151–8.

41. Mendelson WB. Efficacy of melatonin as a hypnotic agent. J Biol Rhythms 1997;12(6):651–6.

42. Zhdanova I, Wurtman RJ, Wagstaff J. Effects of a low dose of melatonin on sleep in children with Angelman syndrome. J Pediatr Endocrinol 1999; 12(1):57–67.

43. Van der Heijden K, Smits MG, Van Someren EJ, et al. Effect of melatonin on sleep, behavior, and cognition in ADHD and chronic sleep-onset insomnia. J Am Acad Child Adolesc Psychiatry 2007;46(2):233–41.

44. Wasdell M, Jan JE, Bomben MM, et al. A randomized, placebo-controlled trial of controlled release melatonin treatment of delayed sleep phase syndrome and impaired sleep maintenance in children with neurodevelopmental disabilities. J Pineal Res 2008;44(1):57–64.

45. Braam W, Didden R, Smits M, et al. Melatonin treatment in individuals with intellectual disability and chronic insomnia: a randomized placebo-controlled study. J Intellect Disabil Res 2008;52(3):256–64.

46. Mayer G, Wang-Weigand S, Roth-Schechter B, et al. Efficacy and safety of 6-month nightly ramelteon administration in adults with chronic primary insomnia. Sleep 2009;32(3):351.

47. Riemann D, Voderholzer U, Cohrs S, et al. Trimipramine in primary insomnia: results of a polysomnographic double-blind controlled study. Pharmacopsychiatry 2002;35(5):165–74.

48. Hohagen F, Montero RF, Weiss E. Treatment of primary insomnia with trimipramine: an alternative to benzodiazepine hypnotics? Eur Arch Psychiatry Clin Neurosci 1994;244(2):65–72.

49. Rodenbeck A, Cohrs S, Jordan W, et al. The sleep-improving effects of doxepin are paralleled by a normalized plasma cortisol secretion in primary insomnia. Psychopharmacology (Berl) 2003;170: 423–8.

50. Hajak G, Rodenbeck A, Adler L, et al. Nocturnal melatonin secretion and sleep after doxepin administration in chronic primary insomnia. Pharmacopsychiatry 1996;29(5):187–92.

51. Hajak G, Rodenbeck A, Voderholzer U, et al. Doxepin in the treatment of primary insomnia: a placebo-controlled, double-blind, polysomnographic study. J Clin Psychiatry 2001;62(6): 453–63.

52. Szabo ST, Thorpy MJ, Mayer G, et al. Neurobiological and immunogenetic aspects of narcolepsy: implications for pharmacotherapy. Sleep Med Rev 2018;43:23–36.

53. Morgenthaler TI, Lee-Chiong T, Alessi C, et al. Standards of Practice Committee of the American Academy of Sleep Medicine. Practice parameters for the clinical evaluation and treatment of circadian rhythm sleep disorders. An American Academy of Sleep Medicine report. Sleep 2007;30(11): 1445–59.

54. Proserpio P, Terzaghi M, Manni R, et al. Drugs used in parasomnia. Sleep Med Clin 2018;13(2): 191–202.

55. Iranzo A. Parasomnias and sleep-related movement disorders in Older adults. Sleep Med Clin 2018;13(1):51–61.

56. Aurora RN, Kristo DA, Bista SR, et al, American Academy of Sleep Medicine. The treatment of restless legs syndrome and periodic limb movement disorder in adults–an update for 2012: practice parameters with an evidence-based systematic review and meta-analyses: an American Academy of Sleep Medicine Clinical Practice Guideline. Sleep 2012;35(8):1039–62.

57. Tobler I, Kopp C, Deboer T, et al. Diazepam-induced changes in sleep: role of the α1 GABAA receptor subtype. Proc Natl Acad Sci U S A 2001;98(11):6464–9.

58. Kopp C, Rudolph U, Low K, et al. Modulation of rhythmic brain activity by diazepam: GABAA receptor subtype and state specificity. Proc Natl Acad Sci U S A 2004;101(10):3674–9.

59. Cope DW, Wulff P, Oberto A, et al. Abolition of zolpidem sensitivity in mice with a point mutation in

the GABAA receptor γ2 subunit. Neuropharmacology 2004;47(1):17–34.

60. Huang MC, Lin HY, Chen CH. Dependence on zolpidem. Psychiatry Clin Neurosci 2007;61:207–8.

61. Cubala WJ, Landowski J. Seizure following sudden zolpidem withdrawal. Prog Neuropsychopharmacol Biol Psychiatry 2007;31:539–40.

62. Hajak G, Müller WE, Wittchen HU, et al. Abuse and dependence potential for the non-benzodiazepine hypnotics zolpidem and zopiclone: a review of case reports and epidemiological data. Addiction 2003;98:1371–8.

63. Verster JC, van de Loo AJ, Moline ML, et al. Middle-of-the-night administration of sleep medication: a critical review of the effects of next morning ability. Curr Drug Saf 2014;9:205–11.

64. Greenblatt DJ, Harmatz JS, Singh NN, et al. Gender differences in pharmacokinetics and pharmacodynamics of zolpidem following sublingual administration. J Clin Pharmacol 2014;54:282–90.

65. Greenblatt DJ, Harmatz JS, von Moltke LL, et al. Comparative kinetics and response to the benzodiazepine agonists triazolam and zolpidem: evaluation of sex-dependent differences. J Pharmacol Exp Ther 2000;293:435–43.

66. Farkas RH, Unger EF, Temple R. Zolpidem and driving impairment–identifying persons at risk. N Engl J Med 2013;369(8):689–91.

67. Greenblatt DJ, Harmatz JS, Roth T, et al. Comparison of pharmacokinetic profiles of zolpidem buffered sublingual tablet and zolpidem oral immediate-release tablet: results from a single-center, single-dose, randomized, open-label crossover study in healthy adults. Clin Ther 2013;35: 604–11.

68. Olubodun JO, Ochs HR, von Moltke LL, et al. Pharmacokinetic properties of zolpidem in elderly and young adults: possible modulation by testosterone in men. Br J Clin Pharmacol 2003;56: 297–304.

69. Pichard L, Gillet G, Bonfils C, et al. Oxidative metabolism of zolpidem by human liver cytochrome P450S. Drug Metab Dispos 1995;23:1253–62.

70. Gillet G. In vitro and in vivo metabolism of zolpidem in three animal species and in man, in Proceedings of the Third International ISSX Meeting Amsterdam.1991.

71. Wolbold R, Klein K, Burk O, et al. Sex is a major determinant of CYP3A4 expression in human liver. Hepatology 2003;38:978–88.

72. Peer CJ, Strope JD, Beedie S, et al. Alcohol and aldehyde dehydrogenases contribute to sex-related differences in clearance of zolpidem in rats. Front Pharmacol 2016;7:260.

73. Aasmoe L, Aarbakke J. Sex-dependent induction of alcohol dehydrogenase activity in rats. Biochem Pharmacol 1999;57:1067–72.

74. Parlesak A, Billinger MH, Bode C, et al. Gastric alcohol dehydrogenase activity in man: influence of gender, age, alcohol consumption and smoking in a caucasian population. Alcohol 2002;37: 388–93.

75. Olivera M, Martınez C, Gervasini G, et al. Effect of common NAT2 variant alleles in the acetylation of the major clonazepam metabolite, 7-aminoclonazepam. Drug Metab Lett 2007;1(1):3–5.

76. Siller N, Egerer G, Weiss J, et al. Prolonged sedation of lorazepam due to absent UGT2B4/2B7 glucuronidation. Arch Toxicol 2014;88(1):179–80.

77. Akutsu T, Kobayashi K, Sakurada K, et al. Identification of human cytochrome p450 isozymes involved in diphenhydramine N-demethylation. Drug Metab Dispos 2007;35(1):72–8.

78. de Leon J, Nikoloff DM. Paradoxical excitation on diphenhydramine may be associated with being a CYP2D6 ultrarapid metabolizer: three case reports. CNS Spectr 2008;13(2):133–5.

79. Saruwatari J, Matsunaga M, Ikeda K, et al. Impact of CYP2D6*10 on H1-antihistamine-induced hypersomnia. Eur J Clin Pharmacol 2006;62(12): 995–1001.

80. Kirchheiner J, Meineke I, Müller G, et al. Contributions of CYP2D6, CYP2C9 and CYP2C19 to the biotransformation of E- and Z-doxepin in healthy volunteers. Pharmacogenetics 2002;12(7):571–80.

81. Mihara K, Kondo T, Suzuki A, et al. Effects of genetic polymorphism of CYP1A2 inductibility on the steady-state plasma concentrations of trazodone and its active metabolite m-chlorophenylpiperazine in depressed Japanese patients. Pharmacol Toxicol 2001;88(5):267–70.

82. Mihara K, Yasui-Furukori N, Kondo T, et al. Relationship between plasma concentrations of trazodone and its active metabolite, m-chlorophenylpiperazine, and its clinical effect in depressed patients. Ther Drug Monit 2002;24(4):563–6.

83. Feuchtl A, Bagli M, Stephan R, et al. Pharmacokinetics of m-chlorophenylpiperazine after intravenous and oral administration in healthy male volunteers: implication for the pharmacodynamic profile. Pharmacopsychiatry 2004;37(4):180–8.

84. Greenblatt DJ, Friedman H, Burstein ES, et al. Trazodone kinetics: effect of age, gender, and obesity. Clin Pharmacol Ther 1987;42(2):193–200.

85. Ishida M, Otani K, Kaneko S, et al. Effects of various factors on steady state plasma concentrations of trazodone and its active metabolite m-chlorophenylpiperazine. Int Clin Psychopharmacol 1995;10(3):143–6.

86. Rotzinger S, Fang J, Coutts RT, et al. Human CYP2D6 and metabolism of m-Chlorophenylpiperazine. Biol Psychiatry 1998;44:1185–91.

87. Zalma A, von Moltke LL, Granda BW, et al. In vitro metabolism of trazodone by CYP3A: inhibition by

ketoconazole and human immunodeficiency viral protease inhibitors. Biol Psychiatry 2000;47(7): 655–61.

88. Staack RF, Maurer HH. Piperazine-derived designer drug 1-3-chlorophenyl)piperazine (mCPP): GC-MS studies on its metabolism and its toxicological detection in rat urine including analytical differentiation from its precursor drugs trazodone and nefazodone. J Anal Toxicol 2003;27:561–8.

89. Tancer ME, Johanson C-E. The subjective effects of MDMA and mCPP amongst moderate MDMA users. Drug Alcohol Depend 2001;65:97–101.

90. Bertilsson L, Dahl ML, Dalén P, et al. Molecular genetics of CYP2D6: clinical relevance with focus on psychotropic drugs. Br J Clin Pharmacol 2002; 53(2):111–22.

91. Thompson MD, Xhaard H, Sakurai T, et al. OX1 and OX2 orexin/hypocretin receptor pharmacogenetics. Front Neurosci 2014;8:57.

92. van Dyck CH, Malison RT, Jacobsen LK, et al. Increased dopamine transporter availability associated with the 9-repeat allele of the SLC6A3 gene. J Nucl Med 2005;46(5):745–51.

93. Ujike H, Harano M, Inada T, et al. Nine- or fewer repeat alleles in VNTR polymorphism of the dopamine transporter gene is a strong risk factor for prolonged methamphetamine psychosis. Pharmacogenomics J 2003;3(4):242–7.

94. Kasparbauer AM, Rujescu D, Riedel M, et al. Methylphenidate effects on brain activity as a function of SLC6A3 genotype and striatal dopamine transporter availability. Neuropsychopharmacology 2015;40(3):736–45.

95. Schacht JP. COMT val158met moderation of dopaminergic drug effects on cognitive function: a critical review. Pharmacogenomics J 2016;16(5): 430–8.

96. Bodenmann S, Xu S, Luhmann UF, et al. Pharmacogenetics of modafinil after sleep loss: catechol-O-methyltransferase genotype modulates waking functions but not recovery sleep. Clin Pharmacol Ther 2009;85(3):296–304.

97. Hamidovic A, Dlugos A, Palmer AA, et al. Catechol-O-methyltransferase val158met genotype modulates sustained attention in both the drug-free state and in response to amphetamine. Psychiatr Genet 2010;20(3):85–92.

98. Dauvilliers Y, Neidhart E, Tafti M. Sexual dimorphism of the catechol-O-methyltransferase gene

in narcolepsy is associated with response to modafinil. Pharmacogenomics J 2002;2(1):65–8.

99. Hartter S, Korhonen T, Lundgren S, et al. Effect of caffeine intake 12 or 24 hours prior to melatonin intake and CYP1A2*1F polymorphism on CYP1A2 phenotyping by melatonin. Basic Clin Pharmacol Toxicol 2006;99(4):300–4.

100. Braam W, Keijzer H, Struijker Boudier H, et al. CYP1A2 polymorphisms in slow melatonin metabolisers: a possible relationship with autism spectrum disorder? J Intellect Disabil Res 2013;57(11): 993–1000.

101. Bialecka M, Kurzawski M, Klodowska-Duda G, et al. The association of functional catechol-O-methyltransferase haplotypes with risk of Parkinson's disease, levodopa treatment response, and complications. Pharmacogenet Genomics 2008; 18(9):815–21.

102. Kaplan N, Vituri A, Korczyn AD, et al. Sequence variants in SLC6A3, DRD2, and BDNF genes and time to levodopa-induced dyskinesias in Parkinson's disease. J Mol Neurosci 2014;53(2):183–8.

103. Sampaio TF, Dos Santos EUD, de Lima GDC, et al. MAO-B and COMT genetic variations associated with levodopa treatment response in patients with Parkinson's disease. J Clin Pharmacol 2018;58(7): 920–6.

104. Cheshire P, Bertram K, Ling H, et al. Influence of single nucleotide polymorphisms in COMT, MAO-A and BDNF genes on dyskinesias and levodopa use in Parkinson's disease. Neurodegener Dis 2014;13(1):24–8.

105. Kaye CM, Nicholls B. Clinical pharmacokinetics of ropinirole. Clin Pharmacokinet 2000;39(4):243–54.

106. Agundez JAG, García-Martın E, Alonso-Navarro H, et al. Anti-Parkinson's disease drugs and pharmacogenetic considerations. Expert Opin Drug Metab Toxicol 2013;9(7):859–74.

107. Becker ML, Visser LE, van Schaik RH, et al. OCT1 polymorphism is associated with response and survival time in anti-Parkinsonian drug users. Neurogenetics 2011;12(1):79–82.

108. Liu Y-Z, Tang B-S, Yan X-X, et al. Association of the DRD2 and DRD3 polymorphisms with response to pramipexole in Parkinson's disease patients. Eur J Clin Pharmacol 2009;65(7):679–83.

109. Xu S, Liu J, Yang X, et al. Association of the DRD2 CAn-STR and DRD3 Ser9Gly polymorphisms with Parkinson's disease and response to dopamine agonists. J Neurol Sci 2017;372:433–8.

Precision Medicine for Idiopathic Hypersomnia

Isabelle Arnulf, MD, PhD*, Smaranda Leu-Semenescu, MD, Pauline Dodet, MD

KEYWORDS

• Hypersomnia • Long sleep time • Drowsiness • GABA • Modafinil • Sodium oxybate

KEY POINTS

• Idiopathic hypersomnia (IH) is characterized by excessive daytime sleepiness despite normal or prolonged sleep.
• New studies insist on the lack of sensitivity, specificity, and reproducibility of multiple sleep latency tests, and the interest of measuring sleep excess on prolonged protocols.
• Cerebrospinal fluid analysis suggests that some patients with resistant central hypersomnia may produce during wakefulness an endogenous peptide binding GABA-A receptors.
• Functional brain imaging supports this concept, with low activity of the medial prefrontal cortex during wakefulness in patients with IH.
• Retrospective and rare placebo-controlled studies illustrate the respective benefit of modafinil, sodium oxybate, pitolisant, mazindol, flumazenil, and clarithromycin in IH treatment.

INTRODUCTION

Idiopathic hypersomnia (IH) is a rare sleep disorder characterized by excessive daytime sleepiness without sleep onset in rapid eye movement [REM] periods [SOREMPs]), despite normal, undisturbed sleep, of normal or prolonged duration. However, this simple definition broadly covers various clinical profiles of patients, which may be captured by different methods of sleep monitoring, and that illustrate the interest of precision medicine in this disorder. Furthermore, IH definitions have suffered from their contrast with narcolepsy type 1, in which several pathognomonic features, including cataplexy, SOREMps, and later cerebrospinal fluid (CSF) hypocretin-1 deficiency define a more homogeneous disorder. To date, there are no definitive biological markers and causes for IH. In addition, the clinical phenotypes and sleep abnormalities (eg, multiple sleep latency test [MSLT] vs long-term monitoring) are heterogeneous. In the past decade, several cohorts have highlighted the lack of sensitivity and long-term reproducibility of the MSLT in patients with IH (and with narcolepsy type 2) and have tried to develop other methods of sleep monitoring to assess patient symptoms more objectively and to define normative values. A major step in identifying the etiology of central hypersomnolence disorders (apart from hypocretin-1 deficiency), was reached when the Atlanta, Georgia, group found indirect evidence that an endogenous hypnotic neurotransmitter when secreted, stimulates GABA-A receptors in some patients with IH (mostly those multiresistant to stimulants). In addition, functional brain imaging suggests that the medial prefrontal cortex of patients with IH is "asleep" when they would otherwise be characterized as awake. Subsequently, there have been formal, placebo-controlled evaluations of

Disclosure Statement: The authors declare that they have no conflicts of interest related to this article. The authors are members of the National Reference Center for Rares Hypersomnias, which receives annuities from the French Health Ministry in order to electively diagnose and treat these patients, as well as to develop medical and social awareness for these disorders, consensus, cohorts and retrospective studies.
National Reference Center for Rare Hypersomnias, Pitie-Salpetriere University Hospital, APHP, and Sorbonne University, 47-83 Boulevard de l'Hôpital, Paris 75013, France
* Corresponding author.
E-mail address: isabelle.arnulf@aphp.fr

Sleep Med Clin 14 (2019) 333–350
https://doi.org/10.1016/j.jsmc.2019.05.007

sleep.theclinics.com

modafinil and clarithromycin in IH, and retrospective series showing the benefit of sodium oxybate, mazindol, flumazenil, and the new pro-histamine stimulant, pitolisant, in IH.

In many textbooks, IH is often described as "what it is not" (eg, it is not a narcolepsy, a mild chronic sleep insufficiency, especially in long sleepers, an upper airway resistance syndrome, a mood disorder with sleepiness, a posttraumatic hypersomnia, a non-REM [NREM] parasomnia with daytime sleepiness). Because IH is a diagnosis of exclusion, these conditions should be first ruled out. The association of IH symptoms with chronic fatigue syndrome/myalgia, attention deficit hyperactivity disorder, and mood disorders raises the potential for overlap with these disorders and the need for more objective measures. In this article, we discuss IH alone and presume that the other hypersomnia disorders have been ruled out by experienced sleep specialists.

HISTORY

Abnormal hypersomnia has been recognized with various terms (idiopathic narcolepsy, NREM narcolepsy, functional, mixed, or harmonious hypersomnia) since the nineteenth century. Bedrich Roth[1] (Prague, Czech Republic) is considered to be the father of the disorder, having described, since the 1940s, a large series of patients suffering from non-narcoleptic daytime sleepiness with sleep drunkenness. Although some patients in this first series likely suffered from sleep apnea, many of them had clinical features suggestive of IH with long sleep time. In the International Classification of Sleep Disorders (ICSD), the disorder was coined as "idiopathic central nervous system hypersomnolence" in 1979. The condition, named 'idiopathic hypersomnia" in 1990,[2] was split between IH with versus without long sleep time in 2005,[3] and later merged together in 2013.[4] There has been more recent debate to split the condition again, to merge narcolepsy type 2 and IH without long sleep time together and to isolate IH with long sleep time as a separate entity. This "coming and going" movement illustrates the difficulty to define clinical phenotypic clusters in IH. Indeed, studies on IH remain scarce especially if one compares with the number of publications on narcolepsy, a rare disorder, and on Kleine-Levin syndrome, a much rarer syndrome (but has some pathognomic clinical features).

EPIDEMIOLOGY OF IDIOPATHIC HYPERSOMNIA

The exact prevalence of IH is unknown, but it is slightly less frequent in expert centers than narcolepsy, suggesting a prevalence of 1 to 2 affected persons for 10,000 inhabitants. The disorder mostly starts during adolescence and early adulthood (**Table 1**). Several series of patients with IH in expert sleep centers indicate that IH affects women (75%) more than men and more frequently persons of European origin (see **Table 1**). The familial appearance of this disorder is observed more frequently than in narcolepsy, but no formal study of familial aggregation has been published to date. The IH rarity can be compared with daytime sleepiness associated with long sleep in epidemiologic studies. In the general population, 1.6% of adults reported sleeping more than 9 hours per 24 hours with concomitant distress or daytime impairment.[5] This sample contained more women, more young (18–24 years old) and

---

Table 1
Symptoms in idiopathic hypersomnia

1. Excessive daytime sleepiness
   - Continuous drowsiness/fogginess without naps
   - Single vs repeated daytime naps
   - Brief (eg, <30–60 min) vs prolonged naps
   - Restorative vs nonrestorative naps
   - Irresistible (eg, sleep attacks) vs resistible sleep episodes
   - Hyperactive counterstrategy

2. Nighttime sleep
   - Normal vs long (>10 h) duration (during unrestrained conditions)
   - High vs normal or low sleep efficiency
   - Dream recall: absent ("black out"), normal, excessive
   - Sleep inertia: none, mild, or severe (sleep drunkenness)

3. Associated symptoms
   - Automatic behaviors
   - Trouble focusing
   - Sleep-related hallucinations
   - Sleep paralysis
   - Orthostatic hypotension
   - Raynaud phenomenon
   - Headaches

4. Epidemiology
   - Rare neonatal forms
   - Mostly young adult onset
   - Women > men
   - More evening chronotype

older (>65 years old) subjects, and more unemployed and retired persons than workers in the general population. Cerebrovascular diseases, disease of the central nervous system (mostly mood disorders, 12 times more frequent), heart diseases, and diseases of the musculoskeletal system were on average twice more prevalent in this subcategory. This epidemiologic study highlights the differential diagnoses of IH. The prevalence of *Diagnostic and Statistical Manual of Mental Disorders, Fourth Edition* hypersomnia disorder in this sample was 0.5% (0.4%–0.6%),[5] which suggests that IH is underdiagnosed.

THE SPECTRUM OF SLEEPINESS IN IDIOPATHIC HYPERSOMNIA

Although all patients with IH are sleepy, the quality of daytime sleepiness varies among them. Sleepiness ranges from frequent, brief, irresistible, and restorative naps (as in narcolepsy) to continuous drowsiness, culminating in rare, prolonged, and nonrestorative naps (see **Table 1**). Many patients with IH, particularly those with long sleep time, describe rare if any daytime sleep attacks.[6] When naps are taken, 87% of patients with IH report a nap duration longer than 60 minutes; 52% to 78% consider their naps unrefreshing, to the point that many patients avoid the situation to prevent severe postnapping inertia. Patients with IH often report suffering from a continuous nonimperative sleepiness, which leads them to never feel fully awake during the daytime, to feel "foggy" and lack alertness. In patients with sleep drunkenness, this drowsiness is maximal on awakening and may transiently fade in the evening.[6] Consequently, many patients with IH are more alert in the evening than in the morning.[6] Although the descriptions of sleepiness appear different in IH than in narcolepsy type 1, both groups have on average similar scores on the Epworth sleepiness scale (ESS),[7] and benefit to a similar degree from stimulants such as modafinil, sodium oxybate, and mazindol.[7–9]

Maintaining a hyperactive state can help patients with IH to resist sleepiness.[6] This can include any increased motor activity (eg, standing, walking while learning, speaking continuously) or performing several activities at the same time (eg, writing while listening, listening to an audiobook when doing chores).[6] Some patients with IH have a rapid, continuous speech during their medical appointment, as if they need to be excited to maintain a sufficient alertness. On average, patients describe that they cannot sustain attention for more than 1 hour (vs almost 4 hours in controls), suggesting a cognitive fatigability.[6] This lack of attention can produce automatic behaviors (see **Table 1**). In our clinical practice, however, they are often extremely organized, making "to do lists" (possibly to compensate for sleepiness and forgetfulness) and reacting rapidly and precisely to questions and requests, in sharp contrast to the frequent procrastination and disorganization observed in patients with narcolepsy or attention deficit hyperactivity disorder. Eventually, autonomic symptoms, including orthostatic hypotension, headache, and Raynaud phenomenon are reported by half of patients with IH.

SLEEP DURATION IN IDIOPATHIC HYPERSOMNIA

The profile of the major sleep episode in IH varies from a normal (eg, 7–8 hours) sleep duration, sometimes with frequent awakenings, to a prolonged (eg, 10–15 hours) sleep duration with a high sleep efficiency, which seems more specific to IH. In ICSD-2,[3] IH was divided into 2 types, with and without long sleep time, defined by whether the usual sleep duration was more or less than 10 hours per night. The 2 types were later merged in ICSD-3, because the committee considered that there were not enough data yet to demonstrate that these were different entities. However, a recent clustering analysis in a series of patients in Prague (Czech Republic) found 2 clearly different clusters, with differing nocturnal sleep times, and no clinical difference between patients with IH without long sleep time and those with narcolepsy type 2.[10] The cutoff of 10 hours of nocturnal sleep for "long sleep time" has not been determined by a specific analysis, but is derived from the sleep duration defining a long sleeper (a person needing more than 10 hours of sleep to feel alert during daytime). In IH series, the frequency of patients usually sleeping more than 10 hours varies from 19% to 58% (**Table 2**). The term "long sleep time" in IH refers only to the main sleep period, and does not include any daytime napping periods. Some patients with IH will sleep 9 hours during the night and 3 hours during the day, far exceeding this limit of 10 hours when the 24-hour day is considered. During weekdays, sleep duration for patients with IH is often constrained by the working schedule, and does not exceed 7 to 9 hours, whereas sleep rebound of 10 to 18 hours may occur during the weekend and vacations. Most patients with IH feel that they sleep very deeply through the night. Frequent sleep disruption is atypical in IH, although common in narcolepsy.[2] In patients with IH, sleep mentation also varies, from a complete blackout with no memory of anything between the sleep onset and

Table 2
Demographic and clinical features in various series of patients with idiopathic hypersomnia

Measure	IH (Mixed)	IH without LST	IH with LST
Demographic features			
Age at onset, y	17 ± 9[11]; 17.5–18[45]; 20 [16][44]; 22 ± 9[8]; 22 ± 12[7]	16[16]; 19 ± 7[51]; 22[25]; 22 ± 13[18]; 29 ± 10[10]	16[16]; 21 ± 9[10]; 24[25]
Age at diagnosis, y	29 ± 12[8]; 33 ± 13[7]; 34 ± 12[11]; 34 ± 13[13]; 34 [16][44]; 35[25]	32[16]; 34 ± 13[13]	27[16]; 34 ± 13[13]
Sex ratio, female/male	38[45]; 51[11]; 64[13]; 64[25] 65[44]; 74[7]; 77[27]; 78[8]	42[18]; 44[25]; 49[51]; 60[10,13]; 82[16]	63[25]; 68[13]; 73[10]; 79[16]
European origin, %	93[25]; 100[13]	—	—
Body mass index, kg/m²	24 ± 5[7,13]; 25 [4][11]; 25.4 [6.2][44]; 25–26[45]	22[16]; 25.2 ± 3.6[52]; 26 ± 5[13]	22[16]; 23 ± 4[13]
Circadian score	48 ± 13[13]; 49 ± 8[27]	53 ± 10[13]	44 ± 14[13]
Daytime symptoms			
Score on the Epworth sleepiness scale at diagnosis, 0–24	14–15[25]; 15 ± 4[13]; 16 ± 3[11]; 16 ± 4[7,8]; 17 ± 4[27]; 17 [7][44]	13.4 ± 6.7[54]; 14.1 ± 3.2[53]; 14 ± 3[51]; 15 ± 4[13]; 15.5 ± 4.3[10] 16.5 ± 4.4[52]; 16.5[16]; 17 ± 4[11]; 18 ± 4[7,25]	15 ± 4[7,13]; 16[16]; 16 ± 3[11]; 16 ± 3.2[10]; 16 ± 4[25]
Nap frequency/wk	2.7 ± 2.6[6]	—	—
Average nap duration, h	1.2 ± 0.5[13]; 1.5 ± 0.9[44]	—	—
Total daytime sleep, min	90 ± 56[13]	89 ± 73[18]	
Sleep attacks, %	54[25]	56[25]; 80[10]	75[25]; 27[10]
Long (>30 min) naps, %	51[25]	—	—
Nap longer than 60 min, %	87[11]	—	—
Refreshing short naps, %	25[6]	56[25]	0[25]
Nonrefreshing naps, %	52[6]; 72[44]; 77[25]; 78[11]	8[10]; 45[6]	48[6]; 72[10]
Attention complaint, %	55[6]	—	—
Memory complaint, %	79[6]	—	—
Automatic behaviors, %	58[6]; 61[25]	63[25]	38[25]
Nighttime symptoms			
Usual sleep duration, h	8 [1][44]; 8.4 ± 1.9[25]; 9 ± 2[11]	—	—
Usual sleep time > 10 h, %	19[44]; 30[11]; 58[7]	0[11]	100[11]
Sleep paralysis, %	10[44]; 28[13]; 40[25]	14[16]; 22[53]; 29[13]; 44[25]	19[16]; 23[13]; 25[25]; 27[13]
Hypnagogic hallucination,%	4[44]; 4.5[11]; 24[13]; 43[25]	4[11]; 25[13,53]; 30[16]; 56[25]	5[11]; 23[13]; 27[16]; 38[25]
Difficulty waking up in the morning, %	66[44]; 100[8]	11[25]; 40[10]; 60[16]	75[25]; 77[16]; 96[10]
Sleep drunkenness, %	37[13]; 55[11]; 66[44]	0[10]; 11[25]; 23[13]; 46[11]	36[25]; 50[13]; 70[11]; 58.3[10]
Time to get going in the morning, min	42[25]	7 ± 6[25]	72 ± 62[25]

(continued on next page)

Measure	IH (Mixed)	IH without LST	IH with LST
Comorbidities			
Migraine, %	7–12[25]; 8[11]	—	—
Minor depression, %	14[11]	—	—
HAD depression score	7.1 ± 5 (>controls)[13]	7.5 ± 4.6[13]	6.8 ± 5.4[13]
Orthostatic hypotension, headache, Raynaud, %	46[6]; 50[25]	—	—
Allergy, %	12[29]	—	—
Autoimmune disease, %	4[29]	—	—
Inflammatory disease, %	7[29]	—	—
Heavy alcohol drinker, %	9[55]	—	—
Tobacco smoker, %	20[55]	—	—
Substance use, %	2[55]	—	—

Measures are mean ± SD or %, except for x-y which indicate median or mean values form two different IH groups.
Abbreviations: HAD, hospital anxiety and depression rating scale; IH, idiopathic hypersomnia; LST, long sleep time (>10 h).

offset, to vivid dreams (25% of patients[11]) and "being tired of dreaming too much." Sleep-related hallucinations (4%–43% of patients) and sleep paralysis (10%–40%) are reported in IH series.

SLEEP DRUNKENNESS IS A MAJOR FEATURE IN IDIOPATHIC HYPERSOMNIA

The ability to wake up in the morning for patients with IH varies from an easy awakening (as in narcolepsy) to major sleep inertia characterized by a "sleep drunkenness," which can be the main complaint of the patients with IH. Sleep drunkenness is conceptualized as a state intermediate to sleep and wake. It seems to be an exacerbation of the normal sleep inertia observed in the normal population, especially during postdeprivation sleep rebound, and in delayed sleep phase syndrome.[12] With sleep drunkenness, patients may not awaken without several successive, strong alarm clocks, and still may immediately return to sleep. Confusion, slowness, incoordination, and aggressiveness are described. Many patients with IH with sleep drunkenness report being slow during the first hour after awakening, with a poor sense of time. Parents of teenagers with IH report having to shake the patient or pull them away from the bed, as if they would "try to wake up a dead person." The disability associated with sleep drunkenness contributes to tardiness at work or even losing their job. Many patients need to be awakened by

another person, making them dependent on others to keep their work schedule. Mothers with IH have significant difficulties awakening when their baby cries, needing some assistance for performing their parental duties during the night. Sleep drunkenness, however, is not a consistent finding in IH, with the symptom reported by 37% to 100% of patients, depending on series and on the presence of the "long sleep time" phenotype (see **Table 2**). The symptom is independent from sleep time and the presence or absence of slow wave sleep at the end of the night.[13] Patients with unipolar depression also report difficulties waking up, but compared with IH, this is associated with anhedonia and decreased motivation. The severity of sleep drunkenness makes it more specific to IH. Note that rare patients with narcolepsy with long sleep time (a disorder cumulating symptoms and signs of narcolepsy and of IH with long sleep time) also report sleep drunkenness.[14]

MULTIPLE SLEEP LATENCY TEST IS NORMAL IN MOST CASES OF IDIOPATHIC HYPERSOMNIA WITH LONG SLEEP TIME

A striking example in which the MSLT was normal in spite of obviously excessive sleep time was reported by Voderholzer and colleagues.[15] This 16-year-old boy had a 4-year history of severely increased sleep need, daytime fatigue, and great difficulty waking after 9 hours of nighttime sleep, with hypotonia and dizziness in the morning, and no cataplexy or sleep attacks during daytime. His mean daytime sleep latency was 11 minutes (a normal value) despite previously sleeping for 27 hours during 36 hours of monitoring. During longer-term monitoring, he slept 19 hours 22 minutes per 24 hours (from 11 PM to 6:30 PM the next day, with an 97% sleep efficiency). This extreme case illustrates the contrast between a measure of daytime sleep-onset propensity (MSLT) and a measure of ad libitum sleep (long-term sleep monitoring). Ad libitum sleep, measured over 24 to 48 hours, may better capture the sleep needs of people in absence of sleep restriction. By definition, the MSLT should be performed after unrestricted sleep (which would allow recognizing the long sleepers), but many sleep laboratories set up a maximal waking time (from 6:30 AM to 8 AM) for organization purposes and because the first MSLT should start after a minimum time of 90 minutes (ie, between 8 AM and 9:30 AM).

To determine the sensitivity of the MSLT (mean sleep latency [MSL] ≤ 8 minutes) in patients with IH, one has to compare to a reference standard in reaching the IH diagnosis. Studies have used different approaches, including a clinical assessment of IH with careful exclusion of competing diagnoses,[11] or a clinical assessment combined with objective criterion, including either a minimal sleep time during ad libitum long-term monitoring,[13,16] or an abnormal potentiation of the GABA-A receptor in CSF.[17] In other cases, when the MSL for an MSLT is set as abnormal if ≤ 8 minutes, patients without this criterion are generally classified as suffering from "subjective hypersomnia."[18] The Cambridge (United Kingdom) group showed that among 72 patients who had a typical clinical phenotype of IH, including those without long sleep time, 49% did not fulfill the criteria of an MSL less than 8 minutes.

The Paris (France) group defined patients suffering from IH with long sleep time as sleeping more than 11 hours during ad libitum monitoring of 19 hours (second night and second day) following a habituation first night and a first day with MSLT.[13] In the group with total sleep time longer than 10 hours, as many as 71% did not fulfill the criteria of a MSL less than 8 minutes, of which only 17% had borderline (between 8 and 10 minutes) sleep latencies.[13] When considering all patients with IH (with and without long sleep time), the MSL was less than 8 minutes in 61%, still leaving 39% of patients with IH with normal mean sleep latencies.[13] In the Bologna group (Italy), it was not possible to infer the frequency of normal MSL in patients with IH, because those with mean sleep latencies ≥ 8 minutes were ruled out as suffering

from "subjective hypersomnia."[18] The Montpellier (France) group used a 2-step procedure to set up a minimal sleep time per 32 hours of ad libitum monitoring (first night followed by a day and a second night) leading to a lower limit of 19 hours of sleep per 32 hours in 37 patients with frank clinical symptoms of IH and MSL ≤ 10 minutes.[16] Among 90 patients with clear-cut or probable IH, 29 (67.8%) did not fulfill the criteria of a MSL ≤ 8 minutes, despite more than 19 hours of sleep during the 36-hour procedure. Repeating the MSLT using a modified procedure by interrupting each nap after 1 minute of sleep, which should preserve sleep pressure and decrease the sleep-onset latency, in the same group still resulted in 48 (42%) patients with a MSL >8 minutes.

The Atlanta group identified a new biological marker in the CSF suggestive of potentiating the GABA-A receptor function. In 7 patients with drug-resistant hypersomnia and various initial diagnoses (including long sleeper, narcolepsy type 2, and Kleine-Levin syndrome), the activity at the GABA receptor was increased, despite a MSL greater than 8 minutes in 5 (71%) of 7 patients.[17] In 16 patients with non-narcoleptic, drug-resistant hypersomnia and GABA-A receptor potentiation, 6 (37.5%) of 16 had a normal MSL at the MSLT.[19]

THE IMPORTANCE OF MEASURING LONG SLEEP TIME/SLEEP EXCESS

These results highlight the importance of measures outside the MSLT to capture the IH sleep characteristics. The word hypersomnia comes from the Greek root "hyper" for "excessive" and the Latin root "somnius" for sleep. Thus, the word means "sleep excess," not excessive daytime sleepiness. In IH, sleep excess is best expressed in unrestricted conditions, such as during the weekend, holidays, and in the sleep laboratory, with on average 3 additional hours slept than during weekdays.[6] The duration of spontaneous nighttime sleep time can be measured during unrestrained polysomnography; however, this would not include the daytime sleep time performed during naps. Hence, several groups have developed procedures aimed at assessing the maximum sleep time that can be produced in unrestrained (often boring) conditions, over periods lasting 24 to 48 hours.

To avoid potential post–sleep deprivation rebound, the 3 main procedures include the classic recommendation to visit the sleep laboratory after 1 to 2 weeks without sleep deprivation as assessed by sleep log or actigraphy. However, patients with IH with long sleep time hardly sleep more than 7 to 9 hours during weekdays when they work, still leaving them sleep deprived relative to their daily sleep needs, unless tests are performed after 1 week of vacation with unrestrained sleep. The increased homeostatic need for sleep in patients with IH can be partly alleviated by the 48-hour procedure developed in Paris (France), which includes a habituation night followed by 5-nap MSLT test, during which the patients often sleep, although the MSL is longer than in patients with narcolepsy. Whether home-based studies can replace in-laboratory procedures is questionable, as normative measures have not been established for these conditions.

So far, 3 different procedures have been developed to capture sleep excess (**Fig. 1**; **Table 3**).[13,16,18] One of the procedures (Bologna, Italy) does not include normative measures.[18] The shorter procedure is the Paris (France) procedure (48 hours) and the longest (80 hours, in 2 separated periods of 24 hours and 58 hours, respectively) is the Montpellier (France) procedure.

The Paris procedure lasts a total of 48 hours in the sleep laboratory and is routinely used to evaluate central hypersomnolence in most French expert centers for hypersomnia.[13,14,20] In addition to measures obtained during standard polysomnography, the procedure characterizes the "narcoleptic" phenotype (ie, rapidity to fall asleep during the MSLT and identification of SOR-EMPs), and the "sleep excess" phenotype (measured by the time slept during the second night and day). Patients undergo a first nighttime polysomnography interrupted at 6:30 AM, followed by 5 MSLT starting at 8 AM, and a second night and day ad libitum monitoring, with uninterrupted naps in the morning and afternoon, stopped at 5 PM, which provides an 18-hour-long to 20-hour-long opportunity to sleep (see **Fig. 1**A). In 75 patients with IH undergoing the Paris procedure, the sleep time obtained during the 18-hour long-term monitoring in the sleep laboratory was very similar to the usual sleep time during holidays and weekends in patients, suggesting that the procedure is not a completely artificial measure, disconnected from the real world, but is an objective measure.[6] When measures in patients with IH are contrasted with those of age-matched and sex-matched healthy controls, the cutoff of 11 hours of sleep time has the best sensitivity (72%) and specificity (97%). In contrast, a lower cutoff of 10 hours has a sensitivity of 55% and a specificity of 77%; and a higher cutoff of 11 hours 30 minutes is highly specific (100%) but poorly sensitive (53%).[20] Only 1 in 20 patients with residual sleepiness despite adequately treated sleep apnea syndrome slept more than 11 hours during the same procedure, versus none of the patients with obstructive sleep apnea without residual sleepiness and none of the older controls.[20] Notably, up to 18% of patients with narcolepsy slept longer than 11 hours during the long-term procedure. This form of narcolepsy "with long sleep time" was characterized by less-prevalent cataplexy and was more severe in terms of clinical impairment (with more frequent sleep drunkenness and nonrefreshing naps) compared with patients with narcolepsy without long sleep time.[14]

The Bologna (Italy) procedure lasts 60 hours in total (see **Fig. 1**B), and includes an ad libitum monitoring of sleep during the first 48 hours, followed by an MSLT on the third day.[18] Daytime sleep is not imposed in darkness but is dictated by patient preference. The investigators did note that patients with narcolepsy type 1 slept longer during the daytime than those with narcolepsy type 2 or with IH without long sleep time.

The Montpellier procedure starts with standard polysomnography followed by an MSLT (see

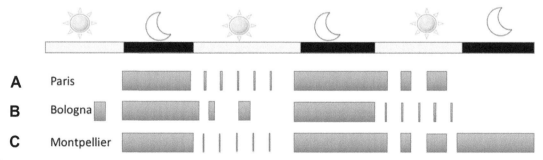

Fig. 1. The various prolonged monitoring procedures used to diagnose IH, when the multiple sleep latency is normal or borderline. A is the Paris (France) procedure, B is the Bologna (France) procedure and C is the Montpellier (France) procedure. Daytime is presented as a yellow bar topped by a sun, night as a dark bar topped by an half moon, over 3 consecutive days and nights (upper line). Blue bars represent sleep periods, either as long sleep episodes (nighttime sleep and long, unrestricted daytime naps) or as brief and restricted naps corresponding to the multiple sleep latency test (presented here as 5 successive brief naps opportunities, lasting 20-34 min in Paris and Bologna and 1 min in Montpellier).

Table 3
Extended sleep-monitoring procedures

Paris procedure[13,14,20]
(48-h protocol)
	Main protocol
	• Night 1: Full polysomnography until 6:30 AM
	• Day 1: 5-nap multiple sleep latency test (MSLT) starting at 8 AM
	• Night 2: ad libitum
	• Day 2: ad libitum until 5 PM
	Notes
	• Dinner at 7 PM on the first night
	• TV, computer, and visits from friends prohibited
	• Books, newspapers, watches, and daylight allowed
	• 2nd night of ad libitum sleep
	  ○ Patient's sleep is not interrupted
	  ○ Patient decides when to sleep and switch off lights
	  ○ Patient decides when to wake up the next day
	• Patients recommended to take 2 naps in a darkened room
	  ○ One in the morning
	  ○ One in the afternoon
	  ○ Stopped after 30 min if patient cannot fall asleep
	  ○ Continued if they do fall asleep until the patient wakes up
	• Meals provided

Bologna procedure[18] (60-h protocol)	Main protocol • Ad libitum sleep for the first 48 h • MSLT on the 3rd day Notes • Patient may move around, read, and watch TV Amount of daytime sleep is determined by the patient

Montpellier procedure[16]
(80-h protocol)
	Main protocol
	• Night 1: Full polysomnography
	• Day 1: 5-nap MSLT
	If borderline sleep latency on the MSLT:
	• Night 2: Full polysomnography
	• Day 2: modified 5-nap MSLT (patient is awoken after 1 min of sleep)
	• Night 3, Day, 3, Night 4: 32-h bed rest procedure – ad libitum sleep
	Notes
	• Amount of daytime sleep is determined by the patient
	• 32-h rest procedure done in darkness
	  ○ Daylight, TV, computer, newspapers, phones, watches, and visits from family and friends prohibited
	  ○ Dim light at 10 lux

Fig. 1C).[16] Then, depending on the clinical assessment and if there is a borderline sleep latency during the MSLT, patients are scheduled for a second procedure lasting 58 hours, beginning with standard polysomnography and followed by a modified MSLT (naps are interrupted after 1 minute of sleep, to avoid decreasing the homeostatic sleep pressure). Sleep is then monitored during a 32-hour bed rest procedure in darkness, including a second night, a second day, and then a third night. Subjects are invited to sleep as long as possible, ad libitum. The investigators determined the sleep duration during the 32-hour bed rest period in 32 patients with typical IH symptoms and mean sleep latencies less than 10 minutes during the first MSLT, and compared it with 21 healthy controls. A cutoff of 19 hours sleep/32 hours of monitoring reached the highest sensitivity (92%) and specificity (86%) to distinguish both groups. When confining the analysis to the first 24 hours of the 32-hour bed rest, a surrogate cutoff of 12 hours of sleep has the highest sensitivity (100%)/specificity (86%).

Each procedure has its advantages (measuring ad libitum, unrestrained sleep during 24–48 hours, ease of implementation) and disadvantages (long duration of testing, availability of normative measures, control of zeitgebers, costs). The 3 laboratories have a long-lasting, unpublished experience with their procedure in other cases (eg, the 48-hour procedure is applied in 20 patients per week in the Paris laboratory during more than 10 years, leading to more than 8000 patients having followed it), which provides some robustness the diagnosis. The cutoffs identified across these procedures, interestingly approximate the cutoffs of 11 to 12 hours during ad libitum sleep that was identified in the ICSD-2 as an alternative criterion of IH with long sleep time in absence of an MSLT less than 8 minutes. Thus, more recent, controlled studies appear to have reached similar conclusions to prior clinical experience from old, uncontrolled studies in expert centers.[21]

MECHANISMS OF IDIOPATHIC HYPERSOMNIA
Triggers

The cause of IH remains unknown. Long sleep time associated with daytime drowsiness can be observed in posttraumatic hypersomnia,[22] post viral hypersomnia, and various hypersomnias associated with neurologic disorders (including tumors of the diencephalon, Prader-Willi syndrome,[23] inflammatory disorders), making it important to rule out these causes (eg, to perform brain MRI, identify head trauma within the last year before hypersomnia onset, and assess for recent viral conversion) before reaching the diagnosis of IH. The onset of IH is usually progressive, making it difficult to identify a trigger. Severe hypersomnia can suddenly occur in the context of a viral infection (eg, Epstein-Barr virus, cytomegalovirus), but the symptoms usually improve after a few months. However, some patients remain sleepy for years. Similarly, some patients have hypersomnia since birth or for decades, but seek medical advice when their life factors change (eg, raising young children, changing of job schedule), which can jeopardize the previous adjustment to what was not considered yet as a disorder.

An Abnormal Sleep Structure?

Many patients with IH sense that their sleep is not normal. In sharp contrast with this feeling, the sleep architecture in IH is classically normal or even "supernormal," with a lower arousal index and higher sleep efficiency than many controls (**Table 4**).[13] The general profile of the sleep architecture in IH is to see NREM and REM sleep in the expected proportions (**Fig. 2**).[24] In various groups of patients with IH, the percentage of N3 has been found to be unchanged,[13,25] decreased,[26] or increased.[11] Notably, some patients with IH display persistent N3 episodes at the end of the night, which is atypical of normal sleepers. The REM sleep has been found to be unchanged,[11,13,25] or increased.[26] This normal or supernormal sleep does not explain why sleep is not restorative of adequate daytime alertness in patients with IH.

Input from Functional Brain Imaging

Recently, the Montreal group performed brain scintigraphy in 13 patients with IH and 16 healthy controls, using single-photon emission computed tomography with ^{99m}Tc-ethyl cysteinate dimer.[27] During wakefulness, patients with IH showed regional cerebral blood flow decreases in medial prefrontal cortex and posterior cingulate cortex and putamen, as well as increases in amygdala and temporo-occipital cortices. Lower regional cerebral blood flow in the medial prefrontal cortex correlated with higher daytime sleepiness, as measured by the ESS and the MSL at the MSLT (**Fig. 3**). The investigators make an interesting parallel between this profile of decreased blood flow in the medial prefrontal cortex in awake patients with IH, which is also seen during NREM stage N2 sleep in healthy subjects.[28] This seminal work suggests that the wakefulness in IH is an intermediate state between wake and sleep, with a seemingly "asleep" medial prefrontal cortex and posterior cingulate cortex and putamen, and compensatory efforts to promote wakefulness from the amygdala and temporo-occipital cortices.

Autoimmunity and Inflammation in Idiopathic Hypersomnia

The rate of comorbid autoimmune disorder is low (4%) in IH, and not different from that of controls.[29] HLA-DQB1*0602 has been examined in many IH series, with frequencies varying from 16% to 31%.[7,8,11,13,30] There was no difference of HLA DQB1*0602 frequency between patients with IH with or without long sleep time,[13] and between patients with IH and healthy controls.[13] Measures of other HLA DRB1 and DQB1 alleles (low resolution) did not identify any differences between 61 patients with IH and 30 controls.[13] In contrast, in our series of 138 patients with IH, the prevalence of inflammatory disorders, allergies, and the incidence of family members with inflammatory disorders was increased in patients compared with controls, suggesting that inflammation may play a role in some cases of IH.[29]

Deficiency of an Arousal System?

Among the arousal systems, in IH there is no deficiency in hypocretin-1 (as there is one in narcolepsy type 1) or in histamine (which is, as hypocretin, released by a single isolated group of neurons).[30] In 29 patients with IH (with or without long sleep time), the hypocretin-1 CSF levels were 307 ± 10 pg/mL.[31] In 26 patients with IH

Table 4
Sleep measures in idiopathic hypersomnia

Measure	IH Unspecified	IH without LST	IH with LST
Multiple sleep latency test (MSLT) and maintenance of wakefulness test (MWT)			
MSL<8 min, %	44[8]; 51[11]; 61[13]	68; 100[13]	11[16]; 29[13]
MSL, min	4.3 ± 2.1[25]; 4.8 [2.5][44]; 5.8–5.9[25]; 7.3 ± 3.2,[27] 7.8 ± 0.5[13]; 8.3 ± 3.1[11] 9.3 ± 3.8[8]	4.3 ± 1.1[25]; 5.6 ± 0.3[13] 5.9 + 1.1[18]; 6.1 ± 3.4[10] 7.9 ± 2.6[11]	3.9 ± 2.4[25]; 8.9 ± 3.5[11] 9.6 ± 0.7[13]; 9.8[16]; 10.2 ± 4[10]
SOREMP, No	0.2 + 0.4[27]	0.2 ± 0.4[10,18]	0.2 ± 0.4[10]
MWT latency, 20 min	12.5–13.5[25]	—	—
Nighttime polysomnography			
Sleep-onset latency, min	7 [9][44]; 12 ± 8[11]; 18–19[25]; 24 ± 21[8]; 31 ± 42[13]	7[16]; 8 ± 7[56] 9 ± 9[52]; 27 ± 27[13]	10[16]; 35 ± 51[13]
REM sleep latency, min	82 [55][44]; 82 ± 48[13]; 106 ± 59[8]	69 ± 42[52]; 74[16] 83 ± 53[13]; 97 ± 53[56]	69[16]; 81 ± 44[13]
Sleep efficiency, % of total sleep time	90 [8][44]; 91 ± 6[13]; 91 ± 15[8]; 92[25]; 93 ± 5[25]; 94 ± 4[11]	87 ± 6[52]; 89 ± 5[25] 89 ± 7[13]; 91 ± 5[56]; 94[16]	92 ± 6[13]; 92.7[16] 96 ± 2[25]
Total sleep time, min	392–420[25]; 454 [62][44] 481 ± 85[8]; 579 ± 90[13]	428 ± 63[52]; 441 ± 23[25] 446[16]; 489 ± 46[56] 517 ± 60[13]	449[16]; 490 ± 50[25]; 633 ± 76[13]
Sleep stages, % of total sleep time			
Stage N1	4 ± 2,[8] 6 [4][44]	4[16]; 11 ± 7[56]	4[16]
Stage N2	50 ± 7[8]; 56 [10][44]	53 ± 8[56]; 56[16]	55[16]
Stage N3	8 ± 5[25]; 15 [8][44]; 18–27[25]; 21 ± 8[13]; 26 ± 8[8]	6 ± 6[25]; 9 ± 8[51]; 21[16]; 21 ± 8[13]	9 ± 6[25]; 20[16]; 21 ± 9[13]
Stage R	18 ± 7[25]; 20–21[25]; 21 ± 5[8] 22 [8][44]; 24 ± 7[13]	14 ± 7[25]; 17[16] 21 ± 5[56]; 23 ± 5[13]	20[16]; 22 ± 4[25] 24 ± 7[13]
Analysis of sleep microstructure			
Arousal index, n/h	9 ± 6[13]; 10 ± 5[8]	10 ± 7[13]	7 ± 4[13]
PLMS index, n/h	1 [4][44]; 3[25]; 3 ± 8[8]; 9 ± 13[13]	0[16]; 1 ± 4[56]; 7 ± 7[52] 11 ± 15[13]	0.3[16]; 5 ± 8[13]
Long-term sleep, ad libitum monitoring			
18 h procedure, min	695 ± 99[13]	635 ± 82[13]	747 ± 82[13]
32 h bed rest procedure, first 24h	—	646[16]	892[16]

Measures are mean ± SD or %, except for those presented as x-y, which represent means or medians from two different IH groups.

Abbreviations: IH, idiopathic hypersomnia; LST, long sleep time; MSL, mean sleep latency; PLMS, periodic leg movements during sleep; REM, rapid eye movement; SOREM, sleep onset in REM period.

without long sleep time, the CSF hypocretin levels were 280.7 ± 14.8 pg/mL.[32] The histamine CSF levels were 161 ± 29.3 pg/mL, a measure in the range of healthy controls.[30] These levels were lower (143.3 ± 28.8 pg/mL) in untreated than treated patients (259.5 ± 94.9 pg/mL), as in narcolepsy and in other disorders associated with daytime sleepiness (including obstructive sleep apnea syndrome), suggesting that histamine is a nonspecific marker of sleepiness.[30] In 6 patients with IH, the CSF levels of melanin-concentrating hormone, which is secreted by the hypothalamus and promotes REM sleep, were 104 ± 26 pg/mL, which was not different from that of healthy controls.[33] Measures of serotonin, norepinephrine,[3-] epinephrine, glutamate, acetylcholine, and their metabolites have been rarely performed in the CSF of patients with IH, with difficult to interpret results when studied.[34] The likelihood that a single bioamine deficiency would specifically affect the

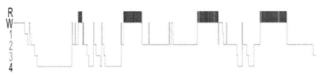

Fig. 2. Hypnogram in a patient with IH (*bottom*), measured during prolonged monitoring (here 18-h long) in Paris (France), compared with a healthy subject (*top*). Sleep is highly efficient, 9 sleep cycles are performed instead of 4, and slow wave sleep is present even during morning sleep. Y axis: R: REM sleep; W: wakefulness; 1, 2, 3, 4: Non REM sleep N1, N2 and N3 (former 3+4 stages).

arousal system alone is low, as these bioamines are released by numerous neuronal systems out of the arousal networks, and are essential for many other brain functions.

Production of an Endogenous Hypnotic Factor?

Recently, the Atlanta group produced convincing evidence that some resistant cases of hypersomnia (including IH, narcolepsy type 2, "long sleepers," and subjective hypersomnia) could result from the inappropriate release of an endogenous hypnotic substance that activates the GABA-A receptors. In support of this hypothesis, the CSF of these patients was applied to GABA-A receptors and was able to displace the normal GABA-A binding. Furthermore, some of these patients benefited from drugs blocking GABA receptors, including flumazenil (commonly used for benzodiazepine overdose) and clarithromycin (an antibiotic that antagonizes the GABA-A receptor).[17,19] The Montpellier group could not reproduce these results in a group of 15 patients with IH.[35]

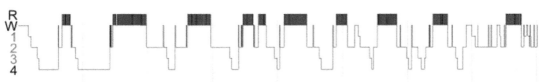

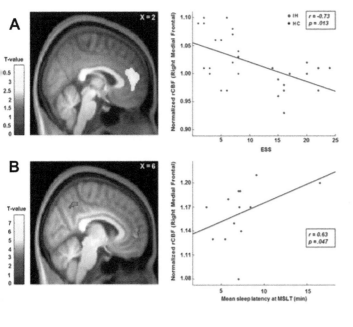

Fig. 3. Decreased regional blood flow in IH (compared with healthy controls [HC], *left*) during brain scintigraphy performed in awake subjects correlates with the level of sleepiness measured by ESS (*A, right*) and by MSLT (*B, right*). rCBF, regional cerebral blood flow. (*From* Boucetta S, Montplaisir J, Zadra A, et al. Altered regional cerebral blood flow in idiopathic hypersomnia. *Sleep* 2017;40(10); with permission.)

Contribution of the Circadian System?

The more frequent evening chronotype in IH,[13] as well as the occasional benefit of evening melatonin to reduce sleep drunkenness,[12,13] has led the Czech group to measure the profile of melatonin secretion over 24 hours in IH.[36] There was a delayed melatonin secretion in 10 patients with IH, which has not been reproduced. In 15 patients with IH, the circadian period length in peripheral skin fibroblast was longer by 0.82 hour than in controls.[37] This finding suggests a genetic contribution of the circadian system in patients with IH. However, of note is that patients with IH do not suffer from delayed sleep phase syndrome, possibly because they try not to shift their sleep onset across nights. This longer circadian period may contribute to the sleep drunkenness observed in these patients.

Animal Models of Idiopathic Hypersomnia?

Animal models have been key for understanding the mechanisms of narcolepsy; however, they have been less helpful in the study of IH. In rodents and feline models, the main arousal systems include histamine and hypocretin neurons in the lateral hypothalamus, norepinephrine, glutamate, and dopamine neurons in the brainstem reticular formation, and acetylcholine neurons in the basal forebrain and in the pedunculopontine nucleus.[38] The selective absence of hypocretin or histamine has not been demonstrated to induce sleep excess in animals. Indeed, mice without hypocretin neurons spend as much time asleep as wild-type mice (both sleep 57% of the 24-hour time period), whereas their periods of wakefulness are fragmented by sleep episodes containing occasional SOREMPs.[39] Mice lacking brain histamine have normal daily sleep duration (accounting for 57% of the time), but are less stimulated by behavioral challenges such as lights off, a new environment, or food delivery.[40] In contrast, a lesion of the dorsal norepinephrine bundle in cats causes a long-lasting, harmonious, severe hypersomnia with 78% of time asleep, with 15% to 27% REM sleep and 73% to 85% NREM sleep.[41] Lesions of the dopamine neurons in the ventral periaqueductal gray matter cause a 20% increase of the daily total sleep time in rats, with proportional increases of NREM and REM sleep.[42]

TREATMENT

No treatment has yet been approved for IH. Current treatment options are based on consensus from professional sleep societies, and, depending on the country, of advice from expert centers, as in France.[43] Many advances in the treatment of narcolepsy have benefited IH, but without the same extent of improvements of symptoms (eg, long, unrefreshing naps and of sleep drunkenness) in patients with IH (**Table 5**).

Preventive Naps

In sharp contrast with narcolepsy, naps (even when brief) are rarely beneficial in IH. Rather, they are often followed by sleep drunkenness and fail to restore adequate alertness. The MSLT is a good test to evaluate their benefit. If naps are beneficial during the MSLT, then they can be recommended as part of a care plan (eg, at school, university, and work). However, knowing that the naps were unrefreshing during the MSLT (eg, "it took me a while to fall asleep and then I was awakened by the nurse, which was horrible") is helpful so that this strategy is not included in the treatment plan.

Reduction and Adaptation of Working Time

There are several adjustments that may help patients remain highly functional at work despite suffering from IH. Accommodations by the employer to allow a patient with IH to begin work at a later hour (eg, to sleep an extra hour in the morning, or not to risk being fired because of lateness), or to work from home (eg, 1 day working home for every 2 days at the work place) can be helpful to patients. Living close to the workplace will reduce the fatigue linked to commuting time and to early awakening. Some patients have developed hyperactivity as a counterstrategy to boost their alertness, such as always being active, speaking frequently, standing, or not resting.[6] Although these activities can be useful counter strategies, patients with IH may need additional rest days separate from vacations, otherwise they may be at risk of exhaustion.

Managing to Wake Up in the Morning

Alarm clocks, phone calls, bright lights, dawn-simulation lights, noises, and pets seem insufficient to assist patients with IH with sleep drunkenness in waking[6] (except in those who have an anxious personality in our experience). Being awoken (and shaken) by another person (parent, spouse, roommate) is efficient, but make patients with IH more dependent on others to achieve adequate awakening.[6] This is particularly problematic for mothers with IH to wake up to prepare their children for school, forcing some families to teach their children

Table 5
Drugs used in idiopathic hypersomnia

Reference	No. Patients	Type of Trial	Benefit	Level of Evidence
Modafinil				
Bastuji and Jouvet,[57] 1988	18	Observational open	Less frequent daily naps in 89%	III
Anderson et al,[11] 2007	39	Observational open	ESS reduction > 4 in 62% Mean ESS reduction: −6 ± 5.4	III
Ali et al,[44] 2009	25	Observational open	72% have a complete (ESS reduction = −9), and 16% a partial response to modafinil	III
Lavault et al,[7] 2011	104	Observational, open, compared with narcolepsy type 1	Over a period of 4.7 y long, mean ESS reduction: −2.6 ± 5.1 in IH, vs −3 ± 5.1 in the narcolepsy group (ITT analysis). Mean efficacy on analogic visual scale: 6.9/10 in IH, vs 6.5/10 in the narcolepsy group	IIb
Philip et al,[46] 2014	14	Randomized, double-blind crossover, vs placebo	In a composite group of patients with IH and patients with narcolepsy, improved driving performance and improved MWT (from 19.7 ± 9.2 min under placebo to 30.8 ± 9.8 min)	Ib
Mayer et al,[45] 2015	33	Randomized, double-blind parallel, vs placebo	Over 3 wk, mean ESS reduction: −6 with modafinil 200 mg/d, vs −1.5 with placebo; CGI improved: −1 point; MWT: + 3 min vs 0 min but not significant	Ib
Methylphenidate				
Ali et al,[44] 2009	40	Observational open	52% have a complete (ESS reduction = −9), and 33% a partial response to modafinil	III
Amphetamine, dextroamphetamine, methamphetamine				
Anderson et al,[11] 2007	11	Observational open	54% are responders (ESS reduction > 4)	III
Ali et al,[44] 2009	20	Observational open	25% are complete (ESS reduction = −9) and 10% partial responders	III
Pemoline				
Ali et al,[44] 2009	7	Observational open	43% are responders	III

(continued on next page)

Table 5
(continued)

Reference	No. Patients	Type of Trial	Benefit	Level of Evidence
Mazindol				
Nittur et al,[9] 2013	37	Observational open	The mean ESS reduction was −4.8 ± 4.7; 84% of patients were responders	III
Sodium oxybate				
Leu-Semenescu et al,[8] 2016	46	Observational open, compared with narcolepsy	The ESS reduction was −3.5 ± 4.5, similar to its effect in narcolepsy type 1 (−3.2 ± 4.2). Sleep drunkenness was improved in 71% these patients	IIb
Pitolisant				
Leu-Semenescu et al,[48] 2014	65	Observational open	36% of patients were responders (ESS reduction > 3)	III
Flumazenil				
Trotti et al,[49] 2016	36	Observational open	68% of patients were responders (mean ESS reduction = 5)	III
Clarithromycin				
Trotti et al,[50] 2014	53	Observational open	34% of patients chose to use it in the long term	III
Trotti et al,[19] 2015	23, with 10 IH	Randomized, double-blind crossover, vs placebo	ESS reduction = −3.9 between clarithromycin and placebo, with −5.4 in the IH group with long sleep time; Improved QoL; unchanged PVT	II

Abbreviations: CGI, clinical general impression; ESS, Epworth sleepiness score; IH, idiopathic hypersomnia; ITT, intention to treat; MWT, maintenance of wakefulness test; PVT, psychomotor vigilance test; QoL, quality of life.

to be more autonomous in their morning preparation.

Reducing Sleep Drunkenness

No drug has been approved for sleep drunkenness. The French expert consensus statement mentions that melatonin at 3 mg (or 2 mg slow-release melatonin) at sleep onset may be useful in some patients with IH to reduce sleep drunkenness.[43] Sodium oxybate (whether as a single dose at sleep onset or split into an evening and a night dose) substantially mitigated sleep drunkenness in a case series from our center.[8] Other strategies include prescribing a dose of a stimulant at bedtime after awakening the patient 1 hour before their usual wakeup time and having them ingest the medication or use a transdermal formulation.[12] Improvement in sleep drunkenness has been reported in individual cases with transdermal and subcutaneous flumazenil, a nicotine patch, and etilefrine (the latter in a patient with comorbid hypotension).[12] Bright light therapy rarely dissipates sleep inertia.[6]

Increasing Daytime Alertness

Modafinil

The various drugs prescribed for IH are shown in **Table 5**. Modafinil was approved from 1994 to 2010 in Europe for IH, until approval was revoked due to the lack of trials by pharmaceutical companies. The mean doses were 367 ± 140 mg in the United States,[44] 400 mg in the United Kingdom,[11] 318 ± 192 mg in France,[7] and 200 mg (fixed dose) in Germany.[45]

In an open, retrospective series in 104 patients with IH and 126 patients with narcolepsy type 1, modafinil was the first-line treatment in 96% to 99% of patients.[7] Similar changes in the ESS were reported between patients with IH and patients with narcolepsy (−2.6 ± 5.1 vs −3 ± 5.1) and a similar benefit as estimated by the patients and clinicians; however, the change in the ESS was lower in patients with IH with long sleep time compared with those without long sleep time. Seventy-two percent of patients with IH reported a benefit of modafinil on their symptoms, similar to patients with narcolepsy type 1.[7] In a randomized, double-blind, placebo-controlled study in 33 patients with IH without long sleep time in Germany, the ESS decreased in patients treated with modafinil.[45] Compared with placebo, modafinil decreased sleepiness significantly but did not significantly improve MSL in the maintenance of wakefulness test. The clinical general impression improved significantly from baseline to the last visit on treatment. In a randomized, placebo-controlled

crossover trial of modafinil 400 mg/d in 13 patients with narcolepsy and 14 patients with IH, modafinil treatment was associated with improved driving simulation results.[46] In this study, MSL on the maintenance of wakefulness test greatly improved from 19.7 ± 9.2 minutes with placebo to 30.8 ± 9.8 minutes with modafinil, but results were not separated by diagnosis. The safety of modafinil was similar between IH and in narcolepsy groups.[7] For these reasons, modafinil is considered first-line treatment in IH.[43]

Methylphenidate and amphetamines

Although methylphenidate is frequently used as a second-line medication in IH, very few data are published in case series, and no controlled study has been performed (see **Table 5**). Methylphenidate was the first-line treatment in IH at the Mayo Clinic (Rochester, MN) until 1998, when modafinil emerged.[44] The mean dose of methylphenidate was 50.9 ± 27.3 mg/d in 61 patients, of whom 40 took as monotherapy. Patients took 3 to 4 doses per day using the immediate release form, but many patients took a combination of immediate and slow-release forms. Twenty-one (52%) patients were considered as complete responders (ESS reduction of −9 points on average), 13 (33%) patients were partial responders (ESS reduction of −6 points on average), and 2 (5%) patients did not respond to the drug. In total, 95% of patients were responders to methylphenidate versus 88% to modafinil ($P = .29$).[44]

The use of dextroamphetamine (35.7 ± 44.4 mg/d), methamphetamine (36 ± 17 mg/d), and combination of amphetamine and dextroamphetamine (79.3 ± 30.6 mg/d) in IH has been reported in the United Kingdom[11] and in the United States,[44] alone or in combination with modafinil or methylphenidate, with 25% to 52% of responders, depending on the criteria used to define responders (see **Table 5**). Pemoline (66.9 ± 36.6 mg/d) was used in 7 patients, with 3 (43%) responders.[44] Mazindol is a pseudo-amphetamine that has been developed for losing weight in obese children and was efficacious in open trials in narcolepsy and in cataplexy.[9] In 37 patients with IH resistant to 2 drugs, the ESS fell from 17 ± 4.4 to 12.5 ± 5.1 under treatment with mazindol (maximum dose in patients 3.6 ± 1.2 mg).[9] The benefit was similar if not larger than in patients with narcolepsy. The last company producing mazindol stopped its production in 2016 for insufficient sales.

Pro-histamine drugs

Pitolisant is a new anti-H3 agonist that blocks the presynaptic reuptake of histamine and increases its release in the brain, which was developed and approved in narcolepsy.[47] Our group has used this medication in 65 patients with IH resistant to 3 other medications and observed a beneficial, alerting effect in one-third of the patients (see **Table 5**).[48] The side effects were rare and benign. They included gastralgia, increased appetite, headache, insomnia, and anxiety.

Sodium oxybate

Sodium oxybate (which stimulates GABA-A receptors in the brain) is approved as a treatment of narcolepsy. Daytime sleepiness is reduced when using 2 doses per night, reduces cataplexy, and improves the dyssomnia. The rationale for using sodium oxybate in IH was not obvious at first, as patients with IH sleep well (instead of suffering from dyssomnia) and are difficult to awaken. However, in a single-center, open-label trial of sodium oxybate in our center of 46 patients with IH with no benefits from modafinil, methylphenidate, and amphetamine (see **Table 4**), sodium oxybate resulted in similar benefits as observed in narcolepsy, even when using a lower dose (a single dose at bedtime).[8] The side effects were similar to those observed in narcolepsy, but more frequent in the IH group. Half of the patients with IH stopped sodium oxybate because of disabling nausea and dizziness.

Reducing Daytime Drowsiness

Flumazenil

Following the discovery of a possible, endogenous peptide enhancing GABA-A transmission in the CSF of several patients with IH, the Atlanta group developed strategies aimed at blocking the GABA-A receptors to counteract the action of such a hypnotic peptide. The first candidate was flumazenil, which is commonly used as an antidote for benzodiazepine intoxication. Intravenous flumazenil has a short half-life, and intravenous continuous infusions of flumazenil (0.38–2 mg) were needed in their first trial to improve the psychomotor vigilance test (PVT) in a series of 7 patients with various (IH, narcolepsy type 2, long sleepers, Kleine-Levin syndrome) hypersomnias.[17] The same group developed sublingual and transdermal forms of flumazenil to avoid the immediate destruction of the drug by the liver. Among 36 patients with IH with treatment-refractory sleepiness, 23 (64%) were initial responders to flumazenil (−5 points on ESS).[49] In the full group of treated patients (which included patients with narcolepsies, IH, subjective hypersomnolence, and sleep apnea with hypersomnolence), flumazenil responders were more often women and subjects with sleep inertia.[49] The most common side effect was

dizziness. Approximately one-third of initial responders discontinued flumazenil for various reasons (eg, tolerance, price).[49]

Clarithromycin

These investigators have also looked for oral drugs that have anti-GABA effects. The antibiotic, penicillin, is known to block the GABA receptors and may induce seizure for this effect. The group found that another common antibiotic, clarithromycin, used as a single morning dosage of 500 to 1000 mg/d, reduced subjective sleepiness (but did not change PVT) in a randomized, crossover, double-blind, placebo-controlled study in patients with IH with CSF evidence of endogenous GABA-A receptor activating peptide (see **Table 5**).[19] Clarithromycin may induce a bad taste, and may expose to changes in vaginal and gut flora (mitigated by the use of probiotics), but it is easily available and inexpensive to try determine if there is a short-term and long-term benefit for a patient with IH. In a longer-term study of clarithromycin in 53 patients with IH, 64% reported initial improvement in subjective sleepiness and 38% elected to continue clarithromycin therapy for the long term.[50]

SUMMARY

IH is a devastating and poorly studied disorder, affecting women more often than men. The disorder has not received sufficient medical attention or adequately powered treatment studies due in part to the rarity of the disorder and difficulties with diagnosis. However, recent advances in precision medicine suggest that the disorder can be better characterized in many patients with the use of prolonged protocols rather than the MSLT. The development of home-based monitoring systems, measuring appropriate surrogates of sleep, may be a future approach to support the IH diagnosis. Standardized approaches to medication treatment have developed. The identification of a benzodiazepinelike endogenous peptide in some patients with IH with stimulant-refractory sleepiness paves the way for treating these patients with benzodiazepine antagonists like flumazenil and clarithromycin. Because the prevalence of IH is close to that of narcolepsy, this should motivate pharmaceutical companies to develop drugs targeted for this disorder.

REFERENCES

1. Roth B. Narcolepsy and hypersomnia. Base (Switzerland): Karger; 1980.
2. American Sleep Disorders Association. The international classification of sleep disorders. Diagnosis

and coding manual 1990. American Academy of Sleep Medicine (Ed) Rochester (MN).

3. American Academy of Sleep Medicine. The international classification of sleep disorders - revised. Chicago: American Academy of Sleep Medicine; 2005.

4. American Academy of Sleep Medicine. The international classification of sleep disorders. 3rd edition. Darien (IL): American Academy of Sleep Medicine; 2014.

5. Ohayon M, Reynolds CI, Dauvilliers Y. Excessive sleep duration and quality of life. Ann Neurol 2013; 73:785–94.

6. Vernet C, Leu-Semenescu S, Buzare M, et al. Subjective symptoms in idiopathic hypersomnia: beyond excessive sleepiness. J Sleep Res 2010; 19(4):525–34.

7. Lavault S, Dauvilliers Y, Drouot X, et al. Benefit and risk of modafinil in idiopathic hypersomnia vs. narcolepsy with cataplexy. Sleep Med 2011;12(6): 550–6.

8. Leu-Semenescu S, Louis P, Arnulf I. Benefits and risk of sodium oxybate in idiopathic hypersomnia versus narcolepsy type 1: a chart review. Sleep Med 2016;17:38–44.

9. Nittur N, Konofal E, Dauvilliers Y, et al. Mazindol in narcolepsy and idiopathic and symptomatic hypersomnia refractory to stimulants: a long-term chart review. Sleep Med 2013;14(1):30–6.

10. Sonka K, Susta M, Billiard M. Narcolepsy with and without cataplexy, idiopathic hypersomnia with and without long sleep time: a cluster analysis. Sleep Med 2015;16(2):225–31.

11. Anderson KN, Pilsworth S, Sharples LD, et al. Idiopathic hypersomnia: a study of 77 cases. Sleep 2007;30:1274–81.

12. Trotti L. Waking up is the hardest thing I do all day: sleep inertia and sleep drunkenness. Sleep Med 2017;35:78–84.

13. Vernet C, Arnulf I. Idiopathic hypersomnia with and without long sleep time: a controlled series of 75 patients. Sleep 2009;32(6):753–9.

14. Vernet C, Arnulf I. Narcolepsy with long sleep time: a specific entity? Sleep 2009;32(9):1229–35.

15. Voderholzer U, Backhaus J, Hornyak M, et al. A 19-h spontaneous sleep period in idiopathic central nervous system hypersomnia. J Sleep Res 1998;7:101–3.

16. Evangelista E, Lopez R, Barateau L, et al. Alternative diagnostic criteria for idiopathic hypersomnia: a 32-hour protocol. Ann Neurol 2018;83(2):235–47.

17. Rye DB, Bliwise DL, Parker K, et al. Modulation of vigilance in the primary hypersomnias by endogenous enhancement of GABAA receptors. Sci Transl Med 2012;4(161):161ra151.

18. Pizza F, Moghadam K, Vandi S, et al. Daytime continuous polysomnography predicts MSLT results in hypersomnias of central origin. J Sleep Res 2013; 22:32–40.

19. Trotti LM, Saini P, Bliwise D, et al. Clarithromycin in γ-aminobutyric acid-related hypersomnolence: a randomized, crossover trial. Ann Neurol 2015;78:454–65.

20. Vernet C, Redolfi S, Attali V, et al. Residual sleepiness in obstructive sleep apnoea: phenotype and related symptoms. Eur Respir J 2011;38(1):98–105.

21. Billiard M, Merle C, Carlander B, et al. Idiopathic hypersomnia. Psychiatry Clin Neurosci 1998;52(2): 125–9.

22. Imbach LL, Valko PO, Li T, et al. Increased sleep need and daytime sleepiness 6 months after traumatic brain injury: a prospective controlled clinical trial. Brain 2015;138(Pt 3):726–35.

23. Ghergan A, Coupaye M, Leu-Semenescu S, et al. Prevalence and phenotype of sleep disorders in 60 adults with Prader-Willi syndrome. Sleep 2017;40. https://doi.org/10.1093/sleep/zsx1162.

24. American Academy of Sleep Medicine. International classification of sleep disorders, 2nd edition: diagnostic and coding manual. Westchester (IL): American Academy of Sleep Medicine; 2005.

25. Bassetti C, Aldrich M. Idiopathic hypersomnia. A series of 42 patients. Brain 1997;120(8):1423–35.

26. Sforza E, Gaudreau H, Petit D, et al. Homeostatic sleep regulation in patients with idiopathic hypersomnia. Clin Neurophysiol 2000;111(2):277–82.

27. Boucetta S, Montplaisir J, Zadra A, et al. Altered regional cerebral blood flow in idiopathic hypersomnia. Sleep 2017;40(10).

28. Dang-Vu T, Desseilles M, Laureys S, et al. Cerebral correlates of delta waves during non-REM sleep revisited. Neuroimage 2005;28:14–21.

29. Barateau L, Lopez R, Arnulf I, et al. Comorbidity between central disorders of hypersomnolence and immune-based disorders. Neurology 2017;88: 93–100.

30. Kanbayashi T, Kodama T, Kondo H, et al. CSF histamine contents in narcolepsy, idiopathic hypersomnia and obstructive sleep apnea syndrome. Sleep 2009; 32(2):181–7.

31. Mignot E, Lammers GJ, Ripley B, et al. The role of cerebrospinal fluid hypocretin measurement in the diagnosis of narcolepsy and other hypersomnias. Arch Neurol 2002;59(10):1553–62.

32. Kanbayashi T, Inoue Y, Chiba S, et al. CSF hypocretin-1 (orexin-A) concentrations in narcolepsy with and without cataplexy and idiopathic hypersomnia. J Sleep Res 2002;11(1):91–3.

33. Peyron C, Valentin F, Bayard S, et al. Melanin concentrating hormone in central hypersomnia. Sleep Med 2011;12:768–72.

34. Montplaisir J, de Champlain J, Young SN, et al. Narcolepsy and idiopathic hypersomnia: biogenic amines and related compounds in CSF. Neurology 1982;32(11):1299–302.

35. Dauvilliers Y, Evangelista E, Lopez R, et al. Absence of γ-aminobutyric acid-a receptor potentiation in

central hypersomnolence disorders. Ann Neurol 2016;80:259–68.

36. Nevsimalova S, Blazejova K, Illnerova H, et al. A contribution to pathophysiology of idiopathic hypersomnia. Suppl Clin Neurophysiol 2000;53: 366–70.

37. Materna L, Halfter H, Heidbreder A, et al. Idiopathic hypersomnia patients revealed longer circadian period length in peripheral skin fibroblasts. Front Neurol 2018;9:424.

38. Saper CB, Scammell TE, Lu J. Hypothalamic regulation of sleep and circadian rhythms. Nature 2005; 437(7063):1257–63.

39. Hara J, Beuckmann CT, Nambu T, et al. Genetic ablation of orexin neurons in mice results in narcolepsy, hypophagia, and obesity. Neuron 2001; 30(2):345–54.

40. Parmentier R, Ohtsu H, Djebbara-Hannas Z, et al. Anatomical, physiological, and pharmacological characteristics of histidine decarboxylase knock-out mice: evidence for the role of brain histamine in behavioral and sleep-wake control. J Neurosci 2002;22(17):7695–711.

41. Petitjean F, Sakai K, Blondaux C, et al. Hypersomnia by isthmic lesion in cat. II. Neurophysiological and pharmacological study. Brain Res 1975;88(3): 439–53 [in French].

42. Lu J, Jhou T, Saper C. Identification of wake-active neurones in the ventral periaqueductal gray matter. J Neurosci 2006;26(1):193–202.

43. Lopez R, Arnulf I, Drouot X, et al. French consensus. Management of patients with hypersomnia: which strategy? Rev Neurol (Paris) 2017;173:8–18.

44. Ali M, Auger R, Slocumb N, et al. Idiopathic hypersomnia: clinical features and response to treatment. J Clin Sleep Med 2009;5:562–8.

45. Mayer G, Benes H, Young P, et al. Modafinil in the treatment of idiopathic hypersomnia without long sleep time—a randomized, double-blind, placebo-controlled study. J Sleep Res 2015;24:74–81.

46. Philip P, Chaufton C, Taillard J, et al. Modafinil improves real driving performance in patients with hypersomnia: a randomized double-blind placebo-controlled crossover clinical trial. Sleep 2014;37(3): 483–7.

47. Dauvilliers Y, Bassetti C, Lammers GJ, et al. Pitolisant versus placebo or modafinil in patients with narcolepsy: a double-blind, randomised trial. Lancet Neurol 2013;12:1068–75.

48. Leu-Semenescu S, Nittur N, Golmard J, et al. Effects of pitolisant, a histamine H3 inverse agonist, in drug resistant idiopathic and symptomatic hypersomnia: a chart review. Sleep Med 2014;15:681–7.

49. Trotti LM, Saini P, Koola C, et al. Flumazenil for the treatment of refractory hypersomnolence: clinical experience with 153 patients. J Clin Sleep Med 2016;12(10):1389–94.

50. Trotti L, Saini P, Freeman A, et al. Improvement in daytime sleepiness with clarithromycin in patients with GABA-related hypersomnia: clinical experience. J Psychopharmacol 2014;28(7):697–702.

51. Ozaki A, Inoue Y, Hayashida K, et al. Quality of life in patients with narcolepsy with cataplexy, narcolepsy without cataplexy, and idiopathic hypersomnia without long sleep time: comparison between patients on psychostimulants, drug-naive patients and the general Japanese population. Sleep Med 2012;13(2):200–6.

52. Pizza F, Ferri R, Poli F, et al. Polysomnographic study of nocturnal sleep in idiopathic hypersomnia without long sleep time. J Sleep Res 2013;22:185–96.

53. Sasai T, Inoue Y, Komada Y, et al. Comparison of clinical characteristics among narcolepsy with and without cataplexy and idiopathic hypersomnia without long sleep time, focusing on HLA-DRB1*1501/DQB1*0602 finding. Sleep Med 2008; 10:961–6.

54. Vignatelli L, D'Alessandro R, Mosconi P, et al. Health-related quality of life in Italian patients with narcolepsy: the SF-36 health survey. Sleep Med 2004;5:467–75.

55. Barateau L, Jaussent I, Lopez R, et al. Smoking, alcohol, drug use, abuse and dependence in narcolepsy and idiopathic hypersomnia: a case-control study. Sleep 2016;39(3):573–80.

56. Takei Y, Komada Y, Namba K, et al. Differences in findings of nocturnal polysomnography and multiple sleep latency test between narcolepsy and idiopathic hypersomnia. Clin Neurophysiol 2012;123: 137–41.

57. Bastuji H, Jouvet M. Successful treatment of idiopathic hypersomnia and narcolepsy with modafinil. Prog Neuropsychopharmacol Biol Psychiatry 1988; 12:695–700.

Precision Medicine in Rapid Eye Movement Sleep Behavior Disorder

Birgit Högl, MD[a], Joan Santamaria, MD[b], Alex Iranzo, MD[b],
Ambra Stefani, MD[a],*

KEYWORDS

- Isolated RBD • Idiopathic RBD • Biomarker • Polysomnography • SINBAR • RWA
- REM sleep without atonia • Prodromal RBD

KEY POINTS

- Diagnosis of isolated RBD needs to be accurate and precise due to its relevance as early phase alpha-synucleinopathy.
- Definite diagnosis requires polysomnography and the quantification of electromyographic activity in the chin and the upper extremities is recommended.
- Biomarkers for neurodegeneration in patients with RBD can be useful to identify patients at risk for short-term conversion or to monitor progression.
- A change in terminology has recently been proposed, as the term (clinically) "isolated RBD" is better in line with current knowledge about the underlying alpha-synuclein pathology of RBD.
- RBD has a gradual onset, with a prodromal phase (rapid eye movement sleep without atonia and/or REM behavioral events) progressing on a continuum over time, to full-blown RBD.

INTRODUCTION

"Precision medicine" has rapidly evolved to be a frequently used term. In the context of rapid eye movement (REM) sleep behavior disorder (RBD) it is also a much needed term. Isolated RBD was formerly seen simply as a parasomnia but is now recognized not only as one of the prodromal manifestations of alpha-synuclein diseases but as by far the most specific marker with an exceedingly high likelihood ratio of 130, if correctly diagnosed with video polysomnography (vPSG).[1,2]

The term "precision medicine" accurately describes how precision is needed in order to make a correct diagnosis of RBD. In the specific field of RBD diagnosis there has been remarkable progress in the 30 years since its first formal description,[3] and the formerly purely qualitative diagnostic criteria have evolved into exact quantitative diagnostic criteria.[2]

In this article, the authors focus in detail on aspects of precision medicine in the context of RBD, namely, conventional PSG and video analysis of night sleep recordings, in particular established and evolving automatic analysis methods. They also discuss whether precision medicine detection of RBD can be improved with other biomarkers beyond vPSG and will consider other diagnostic methods for RBD, which may in the future become relevant to diagnose specifically clinically, still isolated, RBD. Research gaps and

Financial Disclosures: The authors have nothing to disclose.

[a] Department of Neurology, Medical University of Innsbruck, Anichstrasse 35, Innsbruck 6020, Austria; [b] Neurology Service, Multidisciplinary Sleep Unit, Hospital Clinic de Barcelona, Institut D'Investigacions Biomèdiques August Pi i Sunyer, Centro de Investigacion Biomedica en Red de Enfermedades Neurodegenerativas, Calle Villarroel, 170, Barcelona 08036, Spain

* Corresponding author. Sleep Disorders Clinic, Department of Neurology, Medical University of Innsbruck, Anichstrasse 35, Innsbruck 6020, Austria.

E-mail address: ambra.stefani@i-med.ac.at

sleep.theclinics.com

evolving concepts are presented and an outlook for future epidemiologic studies and neuroprotective clinical trials[4] is given.

PRECISION MEDICINE IN CONVENTIONAL POLYSOMNOGRAPHY

In humans, RBD was first categorized and termed in 1986 by Carlos H. Schenck, Scott R. Bundlie, Milton G. Ettinger, and Mark W. Mahowald at the Minneapolis University, USA.[3] From the astute observation of these attentive clinicians, it soon became apparent that patients with RBD not only thrashed around in sleep (presumably acting out their dreams, although this is a chicken and egg situation that is still under debate) but would also have "excessive" electromyography (EMG) activity during REM sleep and "excessive" limb jerking.[3] In 1989 the minimum diagnostic criteria for RBD were formulated by Schenck and colleagues[5] and included "PSG abnormality during REM sleep: elevated submental EMG tone or excessive phasic submental or limb EMG twitching; AND: documentation of abnormal REM sleep behaviors during PSG studies (prominent limb or truncal jerking, complex, vigorous, violent behaviors) or a history thereof."

Although these first minimal diagnostic criteria were based on qualitative assessment ("excessive" for all 3 parameters: EMG tone, phasic twitching, and body jerks), they already condensed remarkably well the hallmarks of RBD.[6] In the first International Classification of Sleep Disorders (ICSD),[7] a diagnosis of RBD required "PSG monitoring to demonstrate excessive augmentation of chin EMG tone, and/or excessive chin or limb phasic EMG twitching and excessive limb or body jerking, complex, vigorous or violent behaviors." Several years later the second edition of the ICSD (ICSD 2)[8] formulated new diagnostic criteria: "presence of REM sleep without atonia (RWA): excessive amounts of sustained or intermittent elevation of submental EMG tone or excessive phasic submental or (upper or lower) limb EMG twitching" was enough to diagnose RBD, along with abnormal sleep-related behaviors.

Today, modern precision medicine with digital PSG recording technology carrying synchronized audiovisual recordings and the availability of well-conducted studies enables us to make an accurate and precise diagnosis of RBD.[9,10] This is necessary to rule out multiple confounders, false negatives, and false positives, which appear if a diagnosis of RBD is based only on sleep history and on questionnaires.[2,11,12] vPSG in the setting of RBD is not only a diagnostic instrument but holds multiple biomarkers of neurodegeneration.[2]

Precise diagnosis in this context is very much needed, not only for quantification but also for evaluation of progression or response to interventions.

Different approaches for quantifying EMG or video abnormalities in RBD have been used and extensively reviewed elsewhere.[2,13–15] Briefly, in conventional PSG for a diagnosis of RBD to be made, the following parameters are analyzed: EMG, electroencephalogram (EEG), and electrooculogram (EOG). The most established for RBD diagnosis are chin EMG and upper extremity EMG. EMG activity can be subclassified into tonic, phasic, or any. In recent years, quantified EMG analysis has been performed for multiple muscles[16] and available cutoffs have been provided.[17,18] Although the combination of chin and upper extremity EMG (flexor digitorum superficialis [FDS]) are the most established recommended forms of recording, a minimum type of recording is based on single channel surface EMG of chin muscle tone.[19] This has the advantage of being simple but in the original version is computed offline.[20]

PRECISION MEDICINE IN VIDEO RECORDING AND ANALYSIS FOR REM SLEEP BEHAVIOR DISORDER

Despite the fact that REM sleep-related behaviors are the key feature of RBD, as reflected in the diagnostic criteria,[21] to date, only a few studies have conducted a detailed and systematic video analysis of movements in patients with RBD.[22–24] These scant data consistently show, nevertheless, that the characteristic complex or violent behaviors represent only the tip of the iceberg, whereas simple, minor, and often distal jerks represent the vast majority of REM behaviors in patients with RBD.[22–24]

Although the diagnosis of RBD is straightforward in the presence of typical RBD movements, there is an area left to interpretation when only many repeated minor jerks or few major (but not complex) movements are present. It is important to point out that only sparse data derived from careful video analysis of normal movements during REM sleep are available. To the authors' knowledge, at the time of writing, only one study has performed a systematic video analysis of movements during REM sleep and this was in 100 healthy adults using contemporary vPSG technology, providing normative values for the first time.[25] Such data are much needed to allow clear differentiation between physiologic and pathologic motor activity during REM sleep, as well as for identifying and defining intermediate stages such as prodromal RBD.[26,27]

Moving forward in the investigation of this gray zone, Sixel-Döring and colleagues[26] introduced the concept of REM sleep behavioral events (RBE) to describe movements that are not considered physiologic as they seem to have a purposeful component but that at the same time cannot be undoubtedly classified as typical RBD behaviors. In a 2-year follow-up study, the same group reported that 38% of patients with RBE developed full-blown RBD over time.[27]

Modern precision medicine using high-definition cameras during vPSG enables recognition and accurate analysis and classification of movements in RBD, including the many minor movements, which can often be seen in these patients. Recently, it has been suggested that this background jerking may prove useful as a quantitative biomarker of RBD.[2] However, future studies are needed to further evaluate this potential new marker of neurodegeneration.

Although disease-modifying medications will hopefully soon become available, current treatments for RBD are only symptomatic, that is, aiming to reduce the number and/or severity of REM-related behaviors and unpleasant dreams. When performing a pharmacologic study investigating symptomatic drugs for RBD, the number and severity of RBD events should be used as primary outcomes. Still, current RBD treatment guidelines are based on (often subjective) reports of efficacy in limited series of patients. The first double-blind, randomized, placebo-controlled study for RBD using RBD events as primary outcome, evaluating the efficacy of nelotanserin, has recently been completed but results are not yet available.[28]

AUTOMATIC ANALYSIS METHODS FOR PRECISION DIAGNOSTICS OF RBD

Automatic analysis of the vPSG studies in RBD is necessary for 2 reasons: (1) it will reduce interrater and intrarater variability that inevitably occur with visual analysis of vPSG signals, and (2) it will allow quantitative measurements in a much easier way, making them more rapid, reliable, repeatable, and appropriate for objectively monitoring the evolution of the disease.

Automatic Electromyogram Analysis

Several systems quantitatively analyze the amount of EMG activity in REM sleep expressing this value in different ways. Most systems exclusively analyze the activity of the mentalis or submentalis muscle[20,29,30] and only one analyzes the mentalis plus the FDS muscles.[31] One way of expressing the amount of EMG activity is the REM atonia index,[19] which can vary from 0 (absent EMG atonia) to 1 (normal EMG atonia). According to one study, an atonia index less than 0.8 suggests RBD. Another form is the suprathreshold REM EMG activity metric (STREAM), which computes the variance of the mentalis EMG activity during 3-second epochs and compares the results in REM sleep to a threshold defined during non-REM sleep.[29] In one study, an STREAM cutoff of 15 identified RBD with 100% sensitivity and 71% specificity.[29] A different approach focused on "short- and long-lasting" EMG activity in 1-second epochs beyond a threshold curve[30] and was reported to differentiate patients with RBD from controls. Finally, the SINBAR-based automatic analysis system[31] used the previously suggested cutoff of 32% for the combination of the mentalis and bilateral FDS muscles[17] and found excellent correlations with the manual scoring of EMG activity in RBD, particularly after manual artifact correction. This software has the additional advantage of being integrated into a commercial PSG recording system. There are no studies comparing the clinical utility of each of these automatic systems in RBD. All these automatic analysis systems need expert human supervision to select each REM sleep episode and exclude artifacts from loose electrode, snoring, movements related to arousals, background noise, or 50 Hz artifacts from the analysis.

Automatic Sleep Stage Scoring and Electroencephalogram Analysis

There are various automatic sleep scoring systems currently packed in several commercial recording systems, but they are less reliable in patients with neurologic diseases than in healthy subjects, because the main elements on which sleep scoring is based can be distorted by the neurologic disease.[32] Identifying REM sleep periods manually may be difficult in some patients with RBD by relying only on the normal sleep stage scoring recommendations. Automatic analysis of the EEG during wake and REM sleep has also been performed in several studies and seems to identify differences in patients with RBD who eventually develop a neurodegenerative disease from those who will not, based on the presence of background theta activity instead of the normal alpha EEG activity. This analysis is, however, hindered by the many EMG, body, eye, and facial movement artifacts that occur during RBD behaviors.

Automatic Analysis of Video Images

There are currently no available systems to automatically analyze the video images in RBD, but this is clearly an area of interest, given the variability in reporting the type, intensity, and duration of the movements patients perform during these RBD behaviors.[2]

CAN PRECISION BE IMPROVED WITH OTHER BIOMARKERS BEYOND POLYSOMNOGRAPHY?

Cumulative data indicate that the isolated form of RBD (iRBD) represents the prodromal stage of those neurodegenerative diseases characterized by alpha-synuclein aggregates in the nervous system, namely Parkinson disease (PD) and dementia with Lewy bodies (DLB).[2,33] Follow-up of patients with iRBD demonstrates the eventual conversion to these synucleinopathies.[34–38] The strongest evidence, however, comes for the histologic demonstration of the pathologic hallmark of PD and DLB: alpha-synuclein deposits in peripheral organs of living individuals with iRBD.[39–44] Biopsies of these organs could complement or in the future perhaps sometimes replace vPSG for the diagnosis of iRBD if they demonstrate very high sensitivity and specificity. Patients with isolated RBD also show clinical, neuroimaging, and electrophysiologic biomarkers that are typical of manifest synucleinopathies (**Box 1**).[2,45] Some of these markers identify patients with high risk of short-term conversion and are able to monitor the neurodegenerative process over time. These biomarkers are very common in iRBD, even in those patients who remain disease free after more than 10 years of follow-up.[46] In principle, biomarkers for neurodegeneration in patients with RBD can be stable or dynamic/progressive, useful to identify patients at risk for conversion or the proximity thereof, or even indicate a risk for conversion into a specific subtype of alpha-synuclein–related disease, whereas others may be useful to monitor the disease progression or turn out to be responsive to treatment.[2] A selection of the many biomarkers that have been identified in iRBD has been reviewed:

- *Alpha-synuclein deposition in peripheral organs.* Aggregates of alpha-synuclein have been detected in the colon, submandibular glands, the labial minor salivary glands, the parotid gland, and the skin of living subjects with iRBD. Such inclusions are very rare in healthy controls and probably represent prodromal PD (**Table 1**).[39–44] This observation highlights that iRBD is an alpha-synucleinopathy per se. Biopsies of these organs have provided moderate to high sensitivity (24%–89%) and high specificity (78%–100%) for the detection of alpha synuclein. However, it still remains to be established which site of the body is the least invasive and most safe, sensitive, and specific for being examined for the detection of alpha-synuclein in iRBD.
- *Mild Parkinsonian signs.* The neurologic examination in subjects with iRBD is normal or identifies subtle motor signs that are not sufficient for making the formal diagnosis of PD. In one study, voice and hypomimia appeared first, followed by rigidity, gait abnormalities and limb bradykinesia, and together with a UPDRS-III score greater than 4 points these features identified prodromal Parkinsonism with 88% sensitivity and 94% specificity 2 years before diagnosis.[47] In the authors experience, the first motor signs that appear are unilateral reduced arm swinging and facial akinesia followed by upper limb bradykinesia and rigidity. Resting tremor is uncommon because most patients develop the akinetic rigid Parkinsonian motor subtype.[48]
- *Asymptomatic cognitive dysfunction.* By definition, patients with iRBD have no relevant cognitive complaints.[33] However, it is common that neuropsychological tests show subclinical impairment in the visuospatial memory, and executive domains.[49,50] These abnormalities worsen over time until cognitive symptoms appear and mild cognitive impairment is diagnosed.[33,51] In most of the cases with mild cognitive impairment the development of dementia occurs within 2 to 4 years. In one patient with iRBD who developed mild cognitive impairment and no dementia, post mortem examination showed widespread Lewy bodies in the brainstem, limbic system and hippocampus sparing the cortex.[52]
- *Hyposmia.* Olfactory tests show that odor identification, discrimination, and detection are frequently impaired in iRBD. Impairment of olfactory identification predicts the development of PD and DLB within a 3- to 5-year timeframe.[53,54] Serial smell tests show that olfactory dysfunction does not deteriorate over time indicating that the evaluation of smell is not useful for monitoring the disease process.[55]
- *Substantia nigra abnormalities.* Neuroimaging tools provide indirect evidence of the characteristic neuropathologic substrate of PD within the substantia nigra: dopaminergic neuronal dysfunction,[56] increased iron content,[57] microglia activation,[58] and loss of dorsolateral hyperintensity.[59] DAT-SPECT demonstrates striatal dopaminergic deficit in about 50% of

---

Box 1
Biomarkers in isolated REM sleep behavior disorder

1. Clinical biomarkers

   1.1. Soft motor signs (hypomimia, reduced arm swinging, limb hypokinesia and bradykinesia, postural sway change)

   1.2. Subtle speech impairment

   1.3. Smell loss

   1.4. Color vision impairment

   1.5. Autonomic abnormalities (constipation, orthostatic hypotension, urine urgency and incontinence, and erectile dysfunction)

   1.6. Depression

   1.7. Apathy

   1.8. Anhedonia

   1.9. No association with excessive daytime sleepiness

2. Neurocognitive markers

   2.1. Impaired visuospatial abilities

   2.2. Impaired attention

   2.3. Impaired executive tasks

   2.4. Impaired memory

   2.5. Difficulties in decision making under ambiguity

   2.6. Pareidolic responses

3. Electrophysiologic markers

   3.1. Electroencephalographic slowing in frontal, temporal, and occipital regions during wakefulness and REM sleep

   3.2. Reduced parasympathetic heart rate variability during wakefulness and sleep

   3.3. Normal autonomic sweat responses

   3.4. Impaired thermal somatosensory function

   3.5. Sudomotor dysfunction

   3.6. Esophageal motor impairment

   3.7. Increased gastrointestinal time and colonic volume

   3.8. Retinal nerve fiber layer thinning

   3.9. Reduced P300 amplitude in the event-related potentials

   3.10. Abnormal vestibular evoked myogenic potentials

4. Neuroimaging markers

   4.1. Dopaminergic denervation of the putamen and caudate nucleus

   4.2. Substantia nigra hyperechogenecity

   4.3. Substantia nigra loss of the dorsolateral nigral hyperintensity

   4.4. Abnormal gradient-recalled-echo susceptibility-weighted imaging of the substantia nigra

   4.5. Substantia nigra microglia activation

   4.6. Basal ganglia connectivity dysfunction

   4.7. Altered connectivity between the left substantia nigra with the left putamen and the right occipital lobe

   4.8. Decreased fractional anisotropy and increased mean diffusivity in the midbrain and pontine nuclei that regulate REM sleep

   4.9. Reduced neuromelanin signal intensity in the coeruleus/subcoeruleus area

4.10. Brainstem raphe hypoechogenicity

4.11. Hyperperfusion in the pons and right hippocampus and hypoperfusion in the frontal lobe

4.12. Abnormal metabolic network characterized by increased activity in the pons, hippocampus, thalamus, cerebellum, and sensorimotor cortex and decreased activity in the occipital, parietal, and temporal cortices and the middle cingulate

4.13. Increased gray matter density in the hippocampus

4.14. Decreased gray matter thickness in the frontal lobe

4.15. Decreased cardiac ^{123}I-MBIG scintigraphy in the heart

4.16. Cholinergic denervation in the colon

4.17. Noradrenergic denervation in the thalamus

5. Biological markers

5.1. Alpha-synuclein aggregates in the autonomic nerve fibers that innervate the colon, all salivary glands, and skin

5.2. Low cerebrospinal fluid levels of alpha-synuclein

5.3. Reduced intraepidermal nerve fiber density in the skin

5.4. Downregulation of the microRNA 19b

5.5. Reduced mitochondrial complex I in the colon

5.6. Reduced levels of the antioxidant superoxide dismutase in blood cells

5.7. Increased glycolysis in blood cells

5.8. Alterations of the N-glycans structures in the serum

5.9. Decreased postprandial ghrelin response in the serum

5.10. Altered protein expression levels in the serum

5.11. Presence of single nucleotide polymorphisms SCARB2 and MAPT

5.12. Presence of GBA gene variants in the serum

5.13. Absence of LRRK2 gene mutations in the serum

5.14. Genetic variants (KP876057, KP876056, NM_000345.3:c*860T>A, NM_000345.3:c*2320A>T) of the 3′untranslated region (3′UTR) of alpha-synuclein in the serum

5.15. No association with APOE Ɛ4 allele in the serum

5.16. Abundant gut microbes such as *Anaerotruncus* and several *Bacteriodes spp*

5.17. No circadian rhythmicity for clock genes Per2, Bma1, and Nr1d1 in the serum

5.18. Delayed melatonin secretion

Adapted from Perez-Carbonell L, Iranzo A. Clinical aspects of idiopathic RBD. In: Schenck CH, Högl B, Videnovic A, eds. Rapid-eye-movement sleep behavior disorder. Springer; 2019:33–52; with permission.

patients with iRBD, and a reduction of dopamine transporter tracer uptake by more than 25% in the putamen is a marker of short-term conversion to PD and DLB.[56] Sequential DAT-SPECT shows progressive decline of the tracer binding in the putamen, indicating that this tool can monitor nigrostriatal dopaminergic deficit over time.[60]

OUTLOOK: OTHER DIAGNOSTIC METHODS BEYOND POLYSOMNOGRAPHY

Although vPSG is the gold standard for diagnosing RBD, there is clearly a need for alternatives at least for the screening of at-risk populations, given the labor-intensive nature of this diagnostic system, the difficulties of performing PSG screening studies of RBD in relatively large populations and making follow-up measurements of the disease in an ambulatory setting would be attractive.

Actigraphy is very likely one of these alternatives, as has been demonstrated in a recent multicenter study led by the Innsbruck group.[6] Actigraphy, in the hands of sleep disorder experts, has been shown to identify patients with RBD and to differentiate them from other patients with sleep-related movement disorders. The rationale behind this procedure is that the abnormal

Table 1
Identification of phosphorylated alpha-synuclein aggregates in the peripheral organs of subjects with isolated REM sleep behavior disorder and matched controls

Site of Biopsy (Reference Number)	Patients/Controls (n)	Adequate Material Obtained in iRBD (%)	Sensitivity in iRBD (%)	Specificity in iRBD (%)
Colon submucosa[39]	20/22	82	24	100
Submandibular gland[40]	21/25	54	90	100
Minor labial salivary glands[41]	62/33	100	50	97
Parotid gland[42]	1/9	100	100	78
Skin[43]	12/55	100	75	100
Skin[44]	18/20	100	55	100

movements associated with RBD behaviors tend to occur with a characteristic temporal pattern during sleep. First, there are quasiperiodic clusters of motor activity during sleep, coinciding with the presumed occurrence of REM sleep, and second, there is no motor activity during the first hour of nocturnal rest time because REM latency is not shortened in RBD. Such patterns of motor activity in the dominant arm were shown to be different from those encountered in patients with sleep apnea who also have end-of-apnea–related movements and in patients with restless legs syndrome with associated periodic limb movements during sleep. Confronted with condensed recordings from 2-week actigraphy on a computer screen, blinded sleep experts were able to recognize visually characteristic actigraphy patterns with relatively high sensitivity and specificity, confirming that the visual analysis of actigraphy represents an easy, low-cost, and useful screening instrument for RBD that could be readily applied to general population studies. There was an additional advantage of actigraphy: it allowed identification of RBD even in patients who were not aware of the abnormal behaviors—which cannot be identified through questionnaires—as well as identification of the normal motor activity patterns of controls. Therefore, visual analysis of actigraphy is even able to recognize patients with iRBD who are unaware of their symptoms[61] and might be used as a first step to identify iRBD in the general population, to select patients who will undergo vPSG for confirming diagnosis.

Other potential alternatives deal with the ambulatory recording of PSG. Although commercial ambulatory vPSG systems, where patients are studied at home, have been available for some time, they share with laboratory-based vPSG most of the technical complexities. Recently, however, other simplified systems that use new wearable sensors and printed electrode arrays with soft electrodes[62] such as temporary tattoo dry electrode systems have been able to record EEG, EOG, and EMG with a wireless system and clearly differentiate sleep stages in a comfortable nonlaboratory setting. These systems merit being tested in RBD.

EVOLVING CONCEPTS IN THE PRECISION DIAGNOSIS OF RBD: CLINICALLY ISOLATED RBD AND PRODROMAL RBD

Precision medicine in the context of RBD also implies precision and clarity in definitions. Classically, after the first description of RBD as a new form of parasomnia by Schenck and colleagues[63] in 1986, RBD that is not associated with other comorbidities or provoking factors has been defined as idiopathic RBD. In light of the high conversion rates into PD, DLB, and more rarely multiple system atrophy (MSA), the term "cryptogenic RBD" had been proposed as an alternative.[49] However, since then several independent long-term follow-up studies consistently reported that more than 80% of patients with "idiopathic" RBD eventually developed an alpha-synucleinopathy. Consequently, RBD is presently recognized as an early stage alpha-synucleinopathy in most cases.[37,64–66] Moreover, even patients with long-standing RBD who have not converted to alpha-synucleinopathy after a decade or more are likely to be in a preclinical phase of alpha-synucleinopathy,[46,67] as they present markers of neurodegeneration. In addition, vPSG-confirmed RBD has been recognized according to the Movement Disorder Society's (MDS) research criteria for prodromal PD as the marker with the by far highest likelihood ratio (130) of prodromal PD.[1]

In light of these findings, a revision of the terminology has recently been proposed. Because neither idiopathic nor cryptogenic RBD reflect the progression of RBD to alpha-synucleinopathies, the use of the descriptive term "(clinically) isolated" RBD has been introduced.[2] This term implies not only that there is an underlying neurodegenerative process that has not yet led to other clinical signs beyond RBD but also that there is a subsequent phase in which RBD is not clinically isolated anymore, as motor and/or cognitive symptoms will become manifest. The stage of isolated RBD can be considered equivalent to what was previously called idiopathic RBD.[2] The term also does no longer suggest ignorance regarding the pathologic cause of RBD but is better in line with current knowledge about the underlying alpha synuclein pathology or RBD.

Besides terminology changes, new concepts have been described as current technology allows a deeper and more precise analysis of vPSG. An increasing number of studies have reported intermediate conditions between what on one side is considered to be physiologic REM sleep with preserved muscle atonia (with only a few phasic twitches in EMG associated with bursts of rapid eye movements) and on the other side what can be diagnosed as RBD according to the current criteria.[68] Intermediate conditions include the aforementioned REM behavioral events (RBE) and the isolated RWA (iRWA), in the absence of motor or behavioral events allowing diagnosis of full-blown RBD. Patients with iRWA[69] or RBE[26,27] show a gradual increase in EMG activity or RBE over time, and preliminary pilot studies showed that 14% to 38% develop full-blown RBD over time.[27,69] These data suggest that RBD has a gradual onset, with progressive increments in RWA and RBE on a continuum over time, until diagnostic criteria for RBD are fulfilled. Moreover, in a pilot study markers of alpha-synuclein–related neurodegeneration have been reported to be present in subjects with iRWA,[69] further suggesting that a neurodegenerative process is already taking place at this stage. Therefore, the term "prodromal RBD" should be used (in analogy to prodromal PD), indicating a stage of disease in which symptoms and signs of evolving RBD (ie, iRWA and/or RBE) are present, although not yet meeting established diagnostic criteria for full-blown RBD.[2] Further studies are warranted to better characterize prodromal RBD, as well as its natural course and its implications in the context of alpha-synucleinopathy. Nevertheless, currently available literature suggests that screening for prodromal RBD might enable the identification of individuals at risk of neurodegeneration at a very early stage, even before the development of isolated RBD. This

has potential implications for future neuroprotective trials, as discussed later.

NEUROPROTECTION TRIALS IN iRBD

To date no effective medical intervention has been demonstrated to slow down the neurodegenerative process in subjects with manifest PD, DLB, and MSA. One of the possible reasons for failure is that the neurodegeneration is too advanced for intervention by the time of diagnosis, when Parkinsonism and cognitive impairment have already emerged.[70] One can assume that neuroprotective therapies might have their greatest chance of success if given in the prodromal period of a neurodegenerative disease. Therefore, patients with iRBD seem to be an optimal target population for testing neuroprotective agents for preventing the onset of Parkinsonism and cognitive symptoms. Patients with iRBD are waiting for the discovery of such effective neuroprotective therapy. Today, this therapy and the development of a neuroprotective trial are still unmet needs in iRBD. The authors believe that although the development of a neuroprotective trial in iRBD is challenging, it is feasible. Below, some aspects are addressed that should be considered when designing such a trial.

1. RBD must be confirmed by vPSG.
2. Patients must not have relevant motor and cognitive complaints, and mild cognitive impairment should be excluded.
3. A multicenter randomized, double-blind, placebo-controlled trial is desirable.
4. The trial should be informative within a time frame of less than 5 years. At 5 years from the diagnosis of iRBD the estimated risk of phenoconversion to PD and DLB is 30% to 35%. However, it should be noted that pharmaceutical companies sponsoring the trial would certainly prefer a study of 2 to 3 years duration (when in iRBD the global risk of conversion is 10%–20%).
5. For a trial of only few years, the iRBD population to be enrolled should carry high short-term risk markers of conversion, which include abnormal smell identification,[52,54] DAT SPECT showing reduction of the tracer uptake greater than 25% in one or both putamen,[5] and mild Parkinsonian signs.[36]
6. Combining markers of short-term conversion would allow reduction of the sample size. Using this strategy, one study estimated that 158 patients per arm would need to be recruited into a 2-year trial to have 80% power to find a 50% reduction in disease phenoconversion.[71]

7. The primary endpoint should be the reduction of the incidence of PD, DLB, and mild cognitive impairment according to current diagnostic clinical criteria. For this, baseline and serial assessments should be easily transferable between centers and investigators, including (1) clinical history, (2) neurologic examination including motor examination (eg, MDS-UPDRS-III), and (3) cognitive standardized evaluations (eg, MoCA test).

8. Secondary endpoints would be the modification of biomarkers of disease progression. In iRBD, subclinical nigrostriatal dopaminergic deficit and asymptomatic neuropsychological abnormalities are frequent, measurable, and have been shown to progress with time.[51,60] Serial DAT-SPECT and neuropsychological testing (eg, MoCA test) could be used as surrogate markers. An effective therapy in patients should slow or stop the rate of decline of the tracer uptake in the putamen and stabilize neuropsychological function (eg, MoCA test score) compared with placebo. Selecting these 2 secondary endpoints is relevant since cardinal symptoms of PD and DLB are Parkinsonism secondary to nigrostriatal dopaminergic cell dysfunction and dementia. In iRBD, other markers such as olfactory loss, impaired color vision, depression, constipation, and substantia nigra hyperechogenicity do not change with time. Therefore, they are not useful for monitoring disease progression and will not serve as secondary outcomes in a neuroprotective trial in iRBD. It is assumed that PSG holds useful (and potentially treatment-responsive) outcome measures for RBD trials (eg, amounts of tonic, phasic, any EMG activity in certain individual or combinations of muscles),[17] but robust evidence from progression and treatment studies is needed.

9. The synucleinopathies share some complex pathogenic mechanisms responsible for neurodegeneration, such as alpha-synuclein accumulation and spreading from cell to cell, oxidative stress, inflammation, lysosomal impairment, and mitochondrial dysfunction. A drug or a combination of drugs that interfere with the underlying pathologic substrate may be an attractive neuroprotective strategy in iRBD.

10. If the selected drug blockades the neuron-to-neuron prion-like transmission of alpha-synuclein, it would be desirable to select patients with iRBD in whom deposits of alpha-synuclein were identified in a peripheral organ.[72]

Currently, neuroprotective trials in patients with a recent diagnosis of PD are underway and are evaluating the effect of passive immunization with antisynuclein antibodies.[72] It is finally time for a neuroprotective trial in iRBD. Patients, clinicians, and researchers are ready.

REFERENCES

1. Berg D, Postuma RB, Adler CH, et al. MDS research criteria for prodromal Parkinson's disease. Mov Disord 2015;30(12):1600–11.

2. Hogl B, Stefani A, Videnovic A. Idiopathic REM sleep behaviour disorder and neurodegeneration - an update. Nat Rev Neurol 2018;14(1):40–55.

3. Schenck CH, Bundlie SR, Patterson AL, et al. Rapid eye movement sleep behavior disorder. A treatable parasomnia affecting older adults. JAMA 1987; 257(13):1786–9.

4. Schenck CH, Montplaisir JY, Frauscher B, et al. Rapid eye movement sleep behavior disorder: devising controlled active treatment studies for symptomatic and neuroprotective therapy–a consensus statement from the International Rapid Eye Movement Sleep Behavior Disorder Study Group. Sleep Med 2013;14(8):795–806.

5. Schenck CH, Hurwitz TD, Mahowald MW. Normal and abnormal REM sleep regulation: REM sleep behaviour disorder: an update on a series of 96 patients and a review of the world literature. J Sleep Res 1993;2(4):224–31.

6. Lapierre O, Montplaisir J. Polysomnographic features of REM sleep behavior disorder: development of a scoring method. Neurology 1992;42(7): 1371–4.

7. American Sleep Disorders Association. The International classification of sleep disorders : diagnostic and coding manual. Rochester (MN): American Sleep Disorders Association; 1990.

8. American Academy of Sleep Medicine. International classification of sleep disorders; diagnostic and coding manual. 2nd edition. Westchester (IL): American Academy of Sleep Medicine; 2005.

9. Stefani A, Frauscher B, Högl B. Diagnosis of REM sleep behavior disorder. In: Schenck CH, Högl B, Videnovic A, editors. Rapid-eye-movement sleep behavior disorder. Springer International Publishing; 2019.

10. Videnovic A, Högl B. Toward disease modification trials in RBD: challenges and opportunities. In: Schenck CH, Högl B, Videnovic A, editors. Rapid-eye-movement sleep behavior disorder. Springer International Publishing; 2019.

11. Stiasny-Kolster K, Sixel-Doring F, Trenkwalder C, et al. Diagnostic value of the REM sleep behavior disorder screening questionnaire in Parkinson's disease. Sleep Med 2015;16(1):186–9.

12. Mahlknecht P, Seppi K, Frauscher B, et al. Probable RBD and association with neurodegenerative disease markers: a population-based study. Mov Disord 2015;30(10):1417–21.

13. Högl B. Towards a more objective diagnosis of REM Sleep Behavior Disorder. Somnologie (Berl) 2013; 17(2):94–7.

14. Frauscher B, Högl B. Quality control for diagnosis of REM sleep behavior disorder: criteria, questionnaires, video, and polysomnography. In: Videnovic A, Högl B, editors. Disorders of sleep and circadian rhythms in Parkinson's disease. Vienna (Austria): Springer-Verlag Wien; 2015. p. 145–57.

15. Schenck CH, Högl B, Videnovic A, editors. Rapid-eye-movement sleep behavior disorder. Springer International Publishing; 2019.

16. Frauscher B, Iranzo A, Hogl B, et al. Quantification of electromyographic activity during REM sleep in multiple muscles in REM sleep behavior disorder. Sleep 2008;31(5):724–31.

17. Frauscher B, Iranzo A, Gaig C, et al. Normative EMG values during REM sleep for the diagnosis of REM sleep behavior disorder. Sleep 2012;35(6):835–47.

18. McCarter SJ, St Louis EK, Duwell EJ, et al. Diagnostic thresholds for quantitative REM sleep phasic burst duration, phasic and tonic muscle activity, and REM atonia index in REM sleep behavior disorder with and without comorbid obstructive sleep apnea. Sleep 2014;37(10):1649–62.

19. Ferri R, Rundo F, Manconi M, et al. Improved computation of the atonia index in normal controls and patients with REM sleep behavior disorder. Sleep Med 2010;11(9):947–9.

20. Ferri R, Manconi M, Plazzi G, et al. A quantitative statistical analysis of the submentalis muscle EMG amplitude during sleep in normal controls and patients with REM sleep behavior disorder. J Sleep Res 2008;17(1):89–100.

21. American Academy of Sleep Medicine. The international classification of sleep disorders : diagnostic & coding manual (ICSD-3). 3rd edition 2014. Westchester (IL).

22. Frauscher B, Gschliesser V, Brandauer E, et al. The relation between abnormal behaviors and REM sleep microstructure in patients with REM sleep behavior disorder. Sleep Med 2009;10(2):174–81.

23. Frauscher B, Gschliesser V, Brandauer E, et al. Video analysis of motor events in REM sleep behavior disorder. Mov Disord 2007;22(10):1464–70.

24. Manni R, Terzaghi M, Glorioso M. Motor-behavioral episodes in REM sleep behavior disorder and phasic events during REM sleep. Sleep 2009; 32(2):241–5.

25. Stefani A, Gabelia D, Mitterling T, et al. A prospective video-polysomnographic analysis of movements during physiological sleep in 100 healthy sleepers. Sleep 2015;38(9):1479–87.

26. Sixel-Döring F, Trautmann E, Mollenhauer B, et al. Rapid eye movement sleep behavioral events: a new marker for neurodegeneration in early Parkinson disease? Sleep 2014;37(3):431–8.

27. Sixel-Doring F, Zimmermann J, Wegener A, et al. The evolution of REM sleep behavior disorder in early Parkinson disease. Sleep 2016;39(9):1737–42.

28. ClinicalTrials.gov. Study evaluating nelotanserin for treatment of REM sleep behavior disorder in subjects with dementia (DLB or PDD). 2018. Available at: https://clinicaltrials.gov/ct2/show/NCT02708186. Accessed October 23, 2018.

29. Burns JW, Consens FB, Little RJ, et al. EMG variance during polysomnography as an assessment for REM sleep behavior disorder. Sleep 2007; 30(12):1771–8.

30. Mayer G, Kesper K, Ploch T, et al. Quantification of tonic and phasic muscle activity in REM sleep behavior disorder. J Clin Neurophysiol 2008;25(1):48–55.

31. Frauscher B, Gabelia D, Biermayr M, et al. Validation of an integrated software for the detection of rapid eye movement sleep behavior disorder. Sleep 2014;37(10):1663–71.

32. Santamaria J, Hogl B, Trenkwalder C, et al. Scoring sleep in neurological patients: the need for specific considerations. Sleep 2011;34(10):1283–4.

33. Iranzo A, Santamaria J, Tolosa E. Idiopathic rapid eye movement sleep behaviour disorder: diagnosis, management, and the need for neuroprotective interventions. Lancet Neurol 2016;15(4):405–19.

34. Schenck CH, Bundlie SR, Mahowald MW. Delayed emergence of a parkinsonian disorder in 38% of 29 older men initially diagnosed with idiopathic rapid eye movement sleep behaviour disorder. Neurology 1996;46(2):388–93.

35. Iranzo A, Molinuevo JL, Santamaria J, et al. Rapid-eye-movement sleep behaviour disorder as an early marker for a neurodegenerative disorder: a descriptive study. Lancet Neurol 2006;5(7):572–7.

36. Postuma RB, Gagnon JF, Bertrand JA, et al. Parkinson risk in idiopathic REM sleep behavior disorder preparing for neuroprotective trials. Neurology 2015;84(11):1104–13.

37. Galbiati A, Verga L, Giora E, et al. The risk of neurodegeneration in REM sleep behavior disorder: a systematic review and meta-analysis of longitudinal studies. Sleep Med Rev 2018;43:37–46.

38. Miyamoto T, Miyamoto M. Phenoconversion from idiopathic rapid eye movement sleep behavior disorder to Lewy body disease. Mov Disord Clin Pract 2018;5(5):506–11.

39. Sprenger FS, Stefanova N, Gelpi E, et al. Enteric nervous system alpha-synuclein immunoreactivity in idiopathic REM sleep behavior disorder. Neurology 2015;85(20):1761–8.

40. Vilas D, Iranzo A, Tolosa E, et al. Assessment of alpha-synuclein in submandibular glands of patients

with idiopathic rapid-eye-movement sleep behaviour disorder: a case-control study. Lancet Neurol 2016;15(7):708–18.

51. Iranzo A, Borrego S, Vilaseca I, et al. alpha-Synuclein aggregates in labial salivary glands of idiopathic rapid eye movement sleep behavior disorder. Sleep 2018;41(8).

52. Fernandez-Arcos A, Vilaseca I, Aldecoa I, et al. Alpha-synuclein aggregates in the parotid gland of idiopathic REM sleep behavior disorder. Sleep Med 2018;52:14–7.

53. Antelmi E, Donadio V, Incensi A, et al. Skin nerve phosphorylated alpha-synuclein deposits in idiopathic REM sleep behavior disorder. Neurology 2017;88(22):2128–31.

54. Doppler K, Jentschke HM, Schulmeyer L, et al. Dermal phospho-alpha-synuclein deposits confirm REM sleep behaviour disorder as prodromal Parkinson's disease. Acta Neuropathol 2017;133(4):535–45.

55. Barber TR, Lawton M, Rolinski M, et al. Prodromal Parkinsonism and neurodegenerative risk stratification in REM sleep behaviour disorder. Sleep 2017;40(8).

56. Iranzo A, Stefani A, Serradell M, et al. Characterization of patients with longstanding idiopathic REM sleep behavior disorder. Neurology 2017;89(3):242–8.

57. Postuma RB, Lang AE, Gagnon JF, et al. How does parkinsonism start? Prodromal parkinsonism motor changes in idiopathic REM sleep behaviour disorder. Brain 2012;135(Pt 6):1860–70.

58. Alibiglou L, Videnovic A, Planetta PJ, et al. Subliminal gait initiation deficits in rapid eye movement sleep behavior disorder: a harbinger of freezing of gait? Mov Disord 2016;31(11):1711–9.

59. Ferini-Strambi L, Di Gioia MR, Castronovo V, et al. Neuropsychological assessment in idiopathic REM sleep behavior disorder (RBD): does the idiopathic form of RBD really exist? Neurology 2004;62(1):41–5.

60. Delazer M, Hogl B, Zamarian L, et al. Decision making and executive functions in REM sleep behavior disorder. Sleep 2012;35(5):667–73.

61. Fantini ML, Farini E, Ortelli P, et al. Longitudinal study of cognitive function in idiopathic REM sleep behavior disorder. Sleep 2011;34(5):619–25.

62. Iranzo A, Gelpi E, Tolosa E, et al. Neuropathology of prodromal Lewy body disease. Mov Disord 2014;29(3):410–5.

63. Postuma RB, Gagnon JF, Vendette M, et al. Olfaction and color vision identify impending neurodegeneration in rapid eye movement sleep behavior disorder. Ann Neurol 2011;69(5):811–8.

64. Mahlknecht P, Iranzo A, Hogl B, et al. Olfactory dysfunction predicts early transition to a Lewy body disease in idiopathic RBD. Neurology 2015;84(7):654–8.

55. Iranzo A, Serradell M, Vilaseca I, et al. Longitudinal assessment of olfactory function in idiopathic REM sleep behavior disorder. Parkinsonism Relat Disord 2013;19(6):600–4.

56. Iranzo A, Santamaria J, Valldeoriola F, et al. Dopamine transporter imaging deficit predicts early transition to synucleinopathy in idiopathic REM sleep behavior disorder. Ann Neurol 2017;82(3):419–28.

57. Iranzo A, Stockner H, Serradell M, et al. Five-year follow-up of substantia nigra echogenicity in idiopathic REM sleep behavior disorder. Mov Disord 2014;29(14):1774–80.

58. Stokholm MG, Iranzo A, Ostergaard K, et al. Assessment of neuroinflammation in patients with idiopathic rapid-eye-movement sleep behaviour disorder: a case-control study. Lancet Neurol 2017;16(10):789–96.

59. De Marzi R, Seppi K, Hogl B, et al. Loss of dorsolateral nigral hyperintensity on 3.0 tesla susceptibility-weighted imaging in idiopathic rapid eye movement sleep behavior disorder. Ann Neurol 2016;79(6):1026–30.

60. Iranzo A, Valldeoriola F, Lomena F, et al. Serial dopamine transporter imaging of nigrostriatal function in patients with idiopathic rapid-eye-movement sleep behaviour disorder: a prospective study. Lancet Neurol 2011;10(9):797–805.

61. Stefani A, Heidbreder A, Brandauer E, et al. Screening for idiopathic REM sleep behavior disorder: usefulness of actigraphy. Sleep 2018;41(6).

62. Shustak S, Inzelberg L, Steinberg S, et al. Home monitoring of sleep with a temporary-tattoo EEG, EOG and EMG electrode array: a feasibility study. J Neural Eng 2018;16(2):026024.

63. Schenck CH, Bundlie SR, Ettinger MG, et al. Chronic behavioral disorders of human REM sleep: a new category of parasomnia. Sleep 1986;9(2):293–308.

64. Iranzo A, Tolosa E, Gelpi E, et al. Neurodegenerative disease status and post-mortem pathology in idiopathic rapid-eye-movement sleep behaviour disorder: an observational cohort study. Lancet Neurol 2013;12(5):443–53.

65. Schenck CH, Boeve BF, Mahowald MW. Delayed emergence of a parkinsonian disorder or dementia in 81% of older men initially diagnosed with idiopathic rapid eye movement sleep behavior disorder: a 16-year update on a previously reported series. Sleep Med 2013;14(8):744–8.

66. Postuma RB, Gagnon JF, Vendette M, et al. Quantifying the risk of neurodegenerative disease in idiopathic REM sleep behavior disorder. Neurology 2009;72(15):1296–300.

67. Yao C, Fereshtehnejad SM, Dawson BK, et al. Longstanding disease-free survival in idiopathic REM

sleep behavior disorder: is neurodegeneration inevitable? Parkinsonism Relat Disord 2018;54:99–102.

68. American Academy of Sleep Medicine. The international classification of sleep disorders : diagnostic and coding manual. 3rd edition. Darien (IL): American Academy of Sleep Medicine; 2014. Rev. ed.

69. Stefani A, Gabelia D, Hogl B, et al. Long-term follow-up investigation of isolated rapid eye movement sleep without atonia without rapid eye movement sleep behavior disorder: a pilot study. J Clin Sleep Med 2015;11(11):1273–9.

70. Lang AE, Espay AJ. Disease modification in Parkinson's disease: current approaches, Challenges, and future considerations. Mov Disord 2018;33(5):660–77.

71. Postuma R, Iranzo A, Hu MT, et al. Risk and predictors of dementia and parkinsonism in idiopathic REM sleep behaviour disorder: a multicentre study. Brain 2019;142(3):744–59.

72. Sardi SP, Cedarbaum JM, Brundin P. Targeted therapies for Parkinson's disease: from Genetics to the clinic. Mov Disord 2018;33(5):684–96.

Non-REM Parasomnia
The Promise of Precision Medicine

Joel Erickson, MD, Bradley V. Vaughn, MD*

KEYWORDS

- NREM parasomnias • Disorders of arousal • Precision medicine • Sleep terrors • Sleepwalking
- Confusional arousals • Sleep related eating disorder

KEY POINTS

- Understanding of the pathogenesis and diagnostic testing for non-REM parasomnias is still being developed.
- Polysomnography, imaging studies, and associated conditions may help to identify biomarkers for diagnosis.
- Disorders of arousal seem to have genetic susceptibility with autosomal-dominant patterns of inheritance and possible associations with HLA genes.
- Targets of precision medicine for treatment of non-REM parasomnias are currently limited to studies of response to cognitive therapies and metabolism of pharmacologic agents.

Precision medicine offers the opportunity to selectively apply diagnostic tools to populations determined at risk based on genetics and biomarkers and then select optimal therapies. Thus, precision medicine depends on the identification of markers that accurately predict susceptibility, prognosis, and treatment response for specific disease processes. In the realm of non-REM (NREM) parasomnias, the field is ripe for further research as both diagnostic and therapeutic evidence has yet to be clearly defined. Currently, most NREM parasomnias are defined phenomenologically by the exhibited behaviors. However, early studies have shown the potential to categorize these disorders by underlying pathophysiologic means and in turn create a better taxonomy to apply the principles of precision medicine. Similarly, parasomnia care may learn from other disciplines that have made inroads into genetic physiologic markers to predict treatment response or side effects from pharmacologic and nonpharmacologic therapies.

BACKGROUND

The term parasomnia relates to undesirable physical events or sensory experiences that occur in association with sleep or with the onset or offset of sleep. NREM parasomnias comprise a group of sleep related behaviors that classically arise during NREM sleep. Many times, these events involve common to bizarre behaviors, including seemingly purposeful movements, mentation, and autonomic output, but also may include the potential for injury. The International Classification of Sleep Disorders, Third Edition, categorizes the NREM parasomnias into disorders of arousal (sleepwalking, sleep terrors, confusional arousals) and sleep-related eating disorder (SRED; **Box 1**).[1]

Typically, NREM parasomnias are considered as a mixture of both wakefulness and NREM sleep. Therefore, patients exhibit features of wakefulness, such as eyes open, complex motor behaviors, and some interaction with the environment, with features of NREM sleep, such as amnesia, decreased awareness, or slowed response times.

Disclosure Statement: The authors have nothing to disclose.
Department of Neurology, University of North Carolina, Chapel Hill, University of North Carolina School of Medicine, CB#7025, Chapel Hill, NC 27599-7025, USA
* Corresponding author.
E-mail address: vaughnb@neurology.unc.edu

Sleep Med Clin 14 (2019) 363–370
https://doi.org/10.1016/j.jsmc.2019.05.002

Box 1
Criteria for diagnosis of NREM parasomnias

Disorders of Arousal (International Classification of Sleep Disorders, Third Edition)

A. Recurrent episodes of incomplete awakening from sleep

B. Inappropriate or absent responsiveness to efforts of others to intervene or redirect the person during the episode.

C. Limited (eg, a single visual scene) or no associated cognition or dream imagery.

D. Partial or complete amnesia for the episode.

E. The disturbance is not better explained by another sleep disorder, mental disorder, medical condition, medication, or substance use.

> *Confusional Arousals*: occur with the patient in bed often start with the individual sitting up in bed and looking about in a confused manner.
>
> *Sleepwalking involves* the individual leaving the bed and walking or even running.
>
> *Sleep Terrors* are often accompanied by a cry or piercing scream, autonomic nervous system output and behavioral manifestations of intense fear.

SRED Criteria (International Classification of Sleep Disorders, Third Edition)

A. Recurrent episodes of dysfunctional eating that occur after an arousal during the main sleep period.

B. The presence of at least one of the following in association with the recurrent episodes of involuntary eating:

1. Consumption of peculiar forms or combinations of food or inedible or toxic substances.

2. Sleep-related injurious or potentially injurious behaviors performed while in pursuit of food or while cooking food.

3. Adverse health consequences from recurrent nocturnal eating.

C. There is partial or complete loss of conscious awareness during the eating episode, with subsequent impaired recall.

D. The disturbance is not better explained by another sleep disorder, mental disorder, medical disorder, medication, or substance use.

From ICSD-3 2014- American Academy of Sleep Medicine: International Classification of Sleep Disorders: Diagnostic & Coding Manual, ICSD-3. 2014, Darien: American Academy of Sleep Medicine, 3; with permission.

Patients may report a memory of vague visual imagery and auditory impressions, but most lack vivid details of the events. These disorders typically arise from the deeper stages of NREM sleep; thus, disorders of arousal are associated with conditions that increase the likelihood of slow wave sleep and arousals. Consequently, the risk of events increases with sleep disruptors including sleep deprivation, stress or other sleep disorders. The International Classification of Sleep Disorders, Third Edition, also cites factors such as change in sleeping environment, change in schedule, and internal stimuli such as distended bladder as precipitants.

EPIDEMIOLOGY

Epidemiologic features, such as age or gender, can give us clues for precision medicine to identify those at classical risk or raise suspicion for patients with atypical parasomnia presentations (**Boxes 2** and **3**). Disorders of arousal are more common in children and young adults, but seem to have no gender difference. Stallman's metaanalysis estimated the prevalence of sleepwalking at approximately 5.0% in children and 1.5% in adults.[2] Although the authors recognize the reliance on subjective reporting, they also recognize this may be underreporting especially in adults. This idea is supported by a study showing that married couples are more likely to report sleepwalking than single individuals.[3]

The peak prevalence of NREM parasomnias occurs in childhood. Petit and colleagues[4] (2015) found in their study of 1940 children that the peak prevalence of sleep terrors occurred at age 1.5 years (34% of children), whereas the peak for sleepwalking occurred at age 10 years (13% of children). One-third of the children who had sleep terrors went on to develop sleepwalking. The decrease in NREM parasomnias as children age into adolescents is also well-documented. Furet and colleagues[5] (2011), studying children age 10 to 18 years over a mean of 4.6 years, found that the incidence of sleep terrors and sleepwalking to remit on follow-up by 100% and 65% respectively.

Sleep-related eating seems to have a peak incidence in young adulthood and is more common in females than males. Santin and colleagues[6] (2014) found a peak age at diagnosis around 39 years but symptoms starting on average 8 years before diagnosis. Winkelman and colleagues[7] (1999) study found the disorder to be more common in individuals with eating disorders (16.7% in an inpatient eating disorder setting vs 8.7% in outpatient eating disorder setting) compared with

---

Box 2
Potential risk factors for disorders of arousal

Age – childhood

Family history of childhood or adolescent parasomnia

Sleep deprivation

Sleep apnea

Hypnotic use –especially short half-life medications

ETOH use

Box 4
Possible biomarkers for risk or diagnosis of disorders of arousal that need further study

Genetic markers

    Chromosome 20q12-q13.12

    HLA DQB1*05:01

Autoimmune – antibodies toward IgLON5 associated with HLA DRB1*10:01 and HLA DQB1*05:01

Physiologic measures

    Slow wave sleep hypersynchrony

    Auditory arousal thresholds from stage N3 sleep

    Impaired TMS inhibition of frontal lobe reflexes

    Functional MRI activation of arousal

---

approximately 4.6% of unselected college students. Thus, the association with concern for weight has been identified as a predisposing risk factor. A portion of these patients have a history of sleepwalking. Schenck and colleagues[8] (1993) estimated, from their case series of 38 individuals referred for SRED, that 70% of individuals met the diagnosis of sleep walking, whereas in Winkelman's series only 10% of those with SRED had a history of sleepwalking.

POSSIBLE BIOMARKERS FOR DIAGNOSIS

The use of diagnostic testing for NREM parasomnias has yet to be fully elucidated; therefore, the list of possible biomarkers is likely to increase (Box 4). Part of this challenge comes from few clear ways to identify and confirm the diagnosis. Currently the gold standard is polysomnographic study (PSG) capturing an event arising from NREM sleep while demonstrating mixed features of wake and NREM sleep (Fig. 1). Additionally, this test assesses for provocative associated conditions or identifies other nocturnal event diagnoses. Fois and colleagues[9] (2015) showed that PSG confirmed parasomnia diagnosis in up to 60% of their study population (n = 124). PSG seemed to be primarily helpful for identifying overlapping diagnoses of unsuspected precipitants. Video of suspected events can be helpful in differentiating parasomnia from other disorders. Video PSG analysis of 184 episodes showed 3 specific

---

Box 3
Risk factors for sleep-related eating

Age – young adult

Gender female

History of eating disorder or being weight conscious

History of NREM parasomnia

Hypnotic medication use

---

motor patterns characterized by increasing intensity and complexity.[10] A separate video analysis study identified 3 principal behavioral patterns: arousal behavior (92% of events), nonagitated motor behavior (72%), and distressed emotional behavior (51%). During this study, parasomnia events primarily arose from stage N3 to N4 (100%) versus epileptic events occurring more during stages N1 and N2 (82%).[11] Using PSG, the onset of NREM parasomnia has been associated with abrupt arousal, usually from stage N3 sleep with expressions of confusion, ambulation, or intense fright captured on video. Typically, there is no overall alteration of sleep architecture or sleep–wake cycle.[12] Increased spontaneous awakening and arousal on electroencephalographic (EEG) monitoring during slow wave sleep is present even on nights without episodes and is not seen in controls.[13] EEG in sleep may show more arousals or an increased cyclic alternating pattern rate and hypersynchronous delta waves. Sleep terrors show increased respiratory and heart rates and sympathetic activation. Chewing motions are observed during episodes of SRED.[14] Evidence shows increased slow wave activity and slow oscillations in EEG patterns before sleepwalking events.[15] A second study showed that these changes primarily happen in the 20 seconds before sleepwalking.[16] Although it is uncommon for parasomnia activity to be captured during PSG, Pilon and colleagues[17] (2008) established a technique that provoked events in nearly 100% of their subjects. In their protocol, subjects with a history of sleepwalking were kept awake through their usual sleep period then allowed to sleep during the day while being recorded. Once the

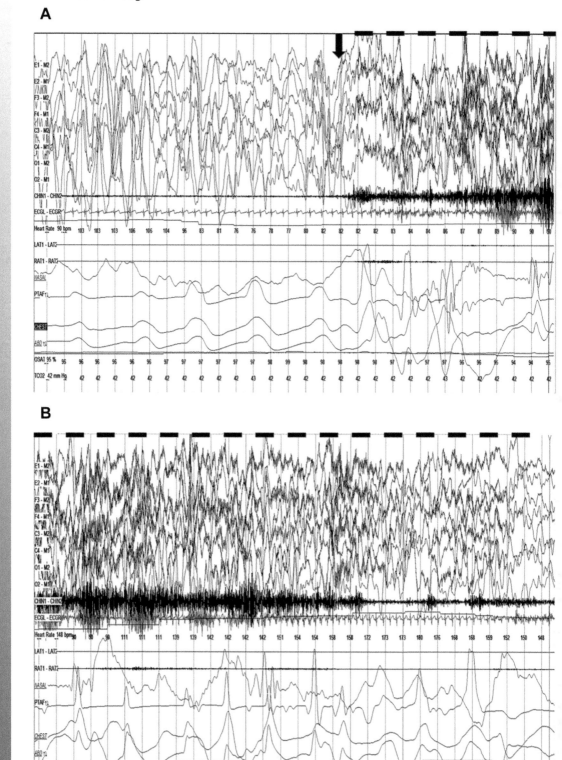

Fig. 1. (*A*, *B*) Onset of a confusional arousal (disorder of arousal event) starting from stage N3 (*arrow*) with continuation of slowing through the arousal (*dashed line*). The patient sat up, seemed to be confused with eyes open, cried out, then returned to sleep.

subjects entered stage N3, an auditory stimulus was introduced causing a partial arousal and subsequent event. This study has yet to be replicated, but does offer a technique that may help to improve diagnostic yield.

Associated conditions may provide additional information to understanding of risk, diagnosis, and possible opportunities for therapy. Disorders of arousal events increase with issues that cause arousal. The most common sleep disorder associated with NREM parasomnias, obstructive sleep apnea (OSA), has also been associated with provoking these parasomnias. Goodwin and colleagues[18] (2004) found that children with a respiratory disturbance index of 1 event per hour or greater were much more likely to have sleepwalking than those with fewer than 1 events per hour (7.0% vs 2.5%, respectively). These children had a higher prevalence of other sleep disorders and learning problems. In adults, Lundetræ and colleagues[19] (2014) found the odds of sleepwalking was higher in severe compared with mild OSA, but were unable to identify a greater risk between OSA and non-OSA in their cohort. These reports raise the issue that disorders of arousal may be a flag for other sleep disorders and that patients with NREM parasomnias may benefit from investigation and treatment of these disorders. Other studies involving imaging tests and more invasive EEG may help to identify additional biomarkers for diagnosis.

Structurally, little evidence exists that the proportions of the brain are different in individuals with disorders of arousals. Heidbreder and colleagues[20] (2017) reported on the structural differences between subjects with NREM parasomnias versus controls using MRI and diffuser tensor imaging. On assessment of gray and white matter volume and density, they found a decreased gray matter volume in the left dorsal posterior cingulate cortex and posterior midcingulate cortex in patients with NREM parasomnia. No other differences were reported, but with only 1 data point authors were unable to conclude the significance.

Stereo-EEG, used during assessment of intractable focal epilepsy patients, showed activation of the motor and central cingulate cortex during NREM parasomnia events with concurrent deactivation of hippocampal and frontal associated cortices.[12] Noninvasive EEG neuroimaging, used to investigate local arousal fluctuations, found local waking activity in the cingulate motor area.[21] Similarly, single-photon emission computed tomography scanning demonstrated that brain perfusion during a sleepwalking episode does not show the same patterns as during sleep

of normal controls.[22] These changes extend to wake conditions after a full night of sleep and after a night of sleep deprivation, showing decreased regional cerebral blood flow bilaterally in inferior temporal gyrus in sleepwalkers versus controls after sleep deprivation.[23]

These studies suggest altered mechanisms of network function in attaining global wakefulness or sleep and thus permitting portions brain to be in incongruent states and allowing mixed function. To investigate this involvement further, Oliviero and colleagues[24] (2007) proposed this may be related to dysfunction of the mechanisms involved in suppressing or allowing arousal. They found the inhibitor reflexes from transcranial magnetic stimulation (TMS) of the frontal lobes in sleepwalkers have an impaired efficiency of inhibitory circuits, such as gamm-aminobutyric acid (GABA)-A neurotransmission, with spared GABA-B neurotransmission during wakefulness. Based on their results, the authors further postulated that concomitant dysfunction of GABA-A and cholinergic pathways predispose the brain to sleepwalking owing to the inability to maintain consolidated slow wave sleep, stop nocturnal movements, and decrease reactivity to sensory stimuli in sleep. They suggested that the impaired inhibition was similar to the immaturity of neural circuits in children, and this finding may correlate with the increased frequency of sleepwalking in childhood.

Disorders of arousal are reported with a number of medical disorders of varied backgrounds including vascular, endocrinologic, and neurologic. A case report discussed an adult de novo case of sleep terrors that the authors related to the presence of a right thalamic lesion on MRI.[25] A case report in Daftary and colleagues[26] (2011) suggested disordered breathing and sleepwalking in a patient with a Chiari I malformation, with symptoms resolving after surgical decompression. In 2018, a case report presented an adult male with new-onset sleepwalking who was found to have mild hyperthyroidism and PSG results showing a decreased percentage of N3 sleep and frequent short awakenings from sleep with associated motor behaviors. Treatment of hyperthyroidism resolved sleepwalking and follow-up PSG showed an increase in total N3 sleep. The authors hypothesized that hyperthyroid arousal intruded into N3 sleep.[27]

Historically, disorders of arousal have been associated with depression and anxiety. However, a study of sleepwalkers found that less than 20% scored in the moderate to severe range of psychopathology on standardized measures of depression and anxiety.[28] Sleep terrors in children do not usually present with psychopathology, but it may play a greater role in adults with sleep terrors.[29]

Some medications seem to incite NREM parasomnias. Zolpidem and other sedative mediations, especially short-acting sedatives, have been reported to increase both sleepwalking events and SRED.[30] This association lends some evidence to possibly impaired arousal mechanisms caused by the medication.

BIOMARKERS FOR SUSCEPTIBILITY

Several factors seem to increase the risk of the disorders of arousal including family history (see **Box 2**). Studies of twins (monozygotic and dizygotic) suggest that genetics play a role in 65% of the cases (International Classification of Sleep Disorders, Third Edition). In 2011, the first genetic locus for sleepwalking reported was at chromosome 20q12-q13.12 and was identified via genome-wide multipoint parametric linkage analysis of a single family of sleepwalkers.[31] Subjects with first-degree relatives with parasomnia have a higher prevalence of NREM parasomnias. In 2015, Petit and colleagues[4] estimated that 47% of children have an NREM parasomnia when 1 parent has a history of sleepwalking and 61% will develop a parasomnia if 2 parents have a history of sleepwalking. These studies suggest an autosomal-dominant pattern of transfer with reduced penetrance, lending to the opportunity for identification of risk for lifetime prevalence, but they do not give clear guidance on who is at risk for NREM parasomnias continuing into adulthood.

Santin and colleagues[6] (2014) found that fewer than 6% of patients with SRED to have a family history of SRED. Correspondingly, eating disorders such as anorexia nervosa seem to run in families. No clear pinpointing genetic pattern has been identified, but some clues suggest as much as 50% of anorexia nervosa is heritable. A genome-wide association study uncovered a connection between anorexia nervosa and a locus overlapping 6 genes on chromosome 12.[32] These findings suggest a mild genetic influence for SRED and thus making genetic testing less likely to help identify patients at risk.

NREM parasomnias have been associated with HLA genes. A retrospective analysis of HLA data from patients with NREM parasomnia (n = 74) and controls showed 75% of subjects had more than 2 different parasomnia types.[33] In this study, HLA DQB1*05:01 was present in 41% of subjects compared with 24% in matched controls. HLA DQB1*0602, which can be found in patients with narcolepsy, was also present in 30% of subjects. The prevalence of HLA genotypes did not differ within the NREM parasomnia type, suggesting a common genetic background.

The presence of HLA associations raises the possibility of autoimmune influences. To date, little research has supported this finding. One exception to this is an overlap parasomnia associated with antibodies toward IgLON5, a neuronal cell adhesion molecule, that has both NREM and REM parasomnia features. IgLON5 disease is a disease of neurodegenerative and autoimmune processes with association to HLA DRB1*10:01 and HLA DQB1*05:01. The disorder is progressive and shows features of tau pathology on autopsy. In a retrospective analysis of 22 subjects with IgLON5 disease, 87% of subjects tested were positive for HLA DQB1*05:01.[34] Clinically these patients show sleep-related vocalizations with movements, as well as complex behaviors and sleep-related breathing disorders. Symptoms usually present at sleep onset, characterized on PSG by undifferentiated NREM or poorly structured N2 sleep followed by normal periods of N2 or N3 NREM sleep.[35]

Adenylate cyclase 5 gene mutations can give us clues into movements and parasomnia movements during sleep. As another potential pathophysiologic avenue, adenylate cyclase 5–related disorders also differ from NREM parasomnias by including dyskinesia that occurs during wakefulness and sleep and sleep architecture disruption.[36]

BIOMARKERS FOR TREATMENT AND TREATMENT RESPONSE

Therapy for disorders of arousal currently rests on 3 major premises: avoidance of provocative factors (sleep deprivation, alcohol, stimuli during sleep), cognitive–behavioral therapy including anticipatory arousals, and reliance on suppression of the arousal by medication. These therapies are focused on decreasing event recurrence and minimizing the risk of injury as the major goal of therapy.

The treatment of disorders of arousal has not been studied systematically. Harris and Grunstein[37] in their 2009 review outlined the essential absence of high-level evidence in the treatment of disorders of arousal. A review by Kierlin and Littner[38] (2011) of the literature of antidepressant therapy for parasomnias revealed some case reports noting medications triggering somnambulism and fewer case reports noting improvement. Since then, no significant clinical trials elucidate the effectiveness of therapies for disorders of arousal but some potential precision medicine targets exist (**Box 5**).

Effect of cognitive–behavioral therapies including anticipatory arousals have been reported to be based on clinical experience. These therapies are traditionally trialed with success being based on report of response. Although anticipatory arousals have not been studied to identify characteristics that predict response, other cognitive–behavioral therapies are searching for such predictive biomarkers. Marwood and colleagues[39] (2018) conducted a metaanalysis of functional MRI data of individuals with depression and anxiety who had a response to psychotherapy. They found that some specific patterns of activation of specific neuronal networks to stimuli before treatment could predict response to therapy. This information opens the potential for the consideration of neural imaging studies to select those individuals who may respond to select psychotherapy or cognitive–behavioral therapies for other conditions such as parasomnias. Similarly, this type of neural network paradigm also suggests that activation studies such as TMS could be a potential biomarker for response to nonpharmacologic as well as pharmacologic therapies.

The pharmacologic treatment of NREM parasomnias focuses primarily on antidepressants and sedative medications. Sedative medications primarily consist of benzodiazepines. Although clinical studies giving clues as to whom may respond to therapy are lacking, these medications offer some application of precision medicine in understanding their metabolism and excretion. This finding is especially true when using pharmacogenetics to identifying those at risk for adverse effects. A prime example of this is clonazepam, which is frequently used to suppress nocturnal events. Clonazepam is extensively metabolized using CYP3A4 or 3A5 to 7-amino-clonazepam and then acetylated to 7-acetamido-clonazepam. The amino clonazepam is a partial agonist and may compete for the GABA receptor binding site. Those individuals who have CYP3A5 protein more rapidly metabolize the CYP3A substrates than those without the protein. Tóth and colleagues[40] (2016), however, found that, when examining patients with schizophrenia or bipolar disorders, the dose requirements for therapeutic concentrations of clonazepam was lower for individuals who had low expression of CYP3A4. These studies have not been replicated in patients with parasomnia, but may be useful in anticipating a target dose. Pharmacogenomic tests to help identify patient's ability to metabolize medications, including other benzodiazepines and antidepressants, are available commercially, but there is ongoing debate as to the clinical usefulness of these tests.

SUMMARY

NREM parasomnias are ripe for investigation to translate precision medicine. Our understanding of the pathogenesis and the key diagnostic testing for NREM parasomnias is still being developed; however, a critical step in making this transition will be to leave the phenomenologic categorization of these disorders and accept a pathophysiologically defined classification scheme. Biomarkers such as hypersynchronous slow waves, impaired TMS inhibition, and possible HLA and genetic links need further investigation and will help us to better understand ways to classify these mysterious events. Once we have better categorization, further research demonstrating the efficacy of our clinical therapies and identifying the key characteristics for optimal therapeutic outcomes will raise the opportunity for tailoring our treatments. We can only look for these studies to help guide us to the potential of the era of precision medicine.

REFERENCES

1. ICSD-3 2014- American Academy of Sleep Medicine. International classification of sleep disorders: diagnostic & coding manual, ICSD-3, vol. 3. Darien (CT): American Academy of Sleep Medicine; 2014.
2. Stallman HM, Kohler M. Prevalence of sleepwalking: a systematic review and meta-analysis. PLoS One 2016;11(11):e0164769.
3. Mume CO. Prevalence of sleepwalking in an adult population. Libyan J Med 2010;5(1):2143.
4. Petit D, Pennestri MH, Paquet J, et al. Childhood sleepwalking and sleep terrors: a longitudinal study of prevalence and familial aggregation. JAMA Pediatr 2015;169(7):653–8.
5. Furet O, Goodwin JL, Quan SF. Incidence and remission of parasomnias among adolescent children in the Tucson children's assessment of sleep apnea (TuCASA) study. Southwest J Pulm Crit Care 2011;2:93–101.
6. Santin J, Mery V, Elso MJ, et al. Sleep-related eating disorder: a descriptive study in Chilean patients. Sleep Med 2014;15(2):163–7.
7. Winkelman JW, Herzog DB, Fava M. The prevalence of sleep-related eating disorder in psychiatric and non-psychiatric populations. Psychol Med 1999;29:1461–6.

8. Schenck CH, Hurwitz TD, O'Connor KA, et al. Additional categories of sleep-related eating disorders and the current status of treatment. Sleep 1993; 16(5):457–66.

9. Fois C, Wright MA, Sechi GP, et al. The utility of polysomnography for the diagnosis of NREM parasomnias: an observational study over 4 years of clinical practice. J Neurol 2015;262(2):385–93.

10. Loddo G, Sessagesimi E, Mignani F, et al. Specific motor patterns of arousal disorders in adults: a video-polysomnographic analysis of 184 episodes. Sleep Med 2018;41:102–9.

11. Derry CP, Harvey AS, Walker MC, et al. NREM arousal parasomnias and their distinction from nocturnal frontal lobe epilepsy: a video EEG analysis. Sleep 2009;32(12):1637–44.

12. Gibbs SA, Proserpio P, Terzaghi M, et al. Sleep-related epileptic behaviors and non-REM-related parasomnias: insights from stereo-EEG. Sleep Med Rev 2016;25:4–20.

13. Gaudreau H, Joncas S, Zadra A, et al. Dynamics of slow-wave activity during the NREM sleep of sleepwalkers and control subjects. Sleep 2000;23: 755–60.

14. Chiaro G, Caletti MT, Provini F. Treatment of sleep-related eating disorder. Curr Treat Options Neurol 2015;17:33.

15. Perrault R, Carrier J, Desautels A, et al. Electroencephalographic slow waves prior to sleepwalking episodes. Sleep Med 2014;15:1468–72.

16. Desjardins M, Carrier J, Lina J, et al. EEG functional connectivity prior to sleepwalking: evidence of interplay between sleep and wakefulness. Sleep 2017; 40(4):zsx024.

17. Pilon M, Montplaisir J, Zadra A. Precipitating factors of somnambulism: impact of sleep deprivation and forced arousals. Neurology 2008;70(24):2274–5.

18. Goodwin JL, Kaemingk KL, Fregosi RF, et al. Parasomnias and sleep disordered breathing in Caucasian and Hispanic children - the Tucson children's assessment of sleep apnea study. BMC Med 2004;2:14.

19. Lundetræ RS, Saxvig IW, Pallesen S, et al. Prevalence of parasomnias in patients with obstructive sleep apnea. A registry-based cross-sectional study. Front Psychol 2018;9:1140.

20. Heidbreder A, Stefani A, Brandauer E, et al. Gray matter abnormalities of the dorsal posterior cingulate in sleep walking. Sleep Med 2017;36:152–5.

21. Januszko P, Niemcewicz S, Gajda T, et al. Sleepwalking episodes are preceded by arousal-related activation in the cingulate motor area: EEG current density imaging. Clin Neurophysiol 2016;127:530–6.

22. Bassetti C, Vella S, Donati F, et al. SPECT during sleepwalking. Lancet 2000;356(9228):484–5.

23. Dang-Vu TT, Zadra A, Labelle MA, et al. Sleep deprivation reveals altered brain perfusion patterns in somnambulism. PLoS One 2015;10(8):e0133474.

24. Oliviero A, Della Marca G, Tonali PA, et al. Functional involvement of cerebral cortex in adult sleepwalking. J Neurol 2007;254(8):1066–72.

25. Di Gennaro G, Autret A, Mascia A, et al. Night terrors associated with thalamic lesion. Clin Neurophysiol 2004;115(11):2489–92.

26. Daftary AS, Walker JM, Farney RJ. NREM sleep parasomnia associated with Chiari I malformation. J Clin Sleep Med 2011;7(5):526–9.

27. Giuliano L, Fatuzzo D, Mainieri G, et al. Adult-onset sleepwalking secondary to hyperthyroidism: polygraphic evidence. J Clin Sleep Med 2018;14(2):285–7.

28. Labelle M, Desautels A, Montplaisir J, et al. Psychopathologic correlates of adult sleepwalking. Sleep Med 2013;14:1348–55.

29. Ohayon MM, Guilleminault C, Priest RG. Night terrors, sleepwalking, and confusional arousals in the general population: their frequency and relationship to other sleep and mental disorders. J Clin Psychiatry 1999;60:268–76.

30. Howell MJ. Parasomnias: an updated review. Neurotherapeutics 2012;9(4):753–75.

31. Licis AK, Desruisseau DM, Yamada KA, et al. Novel genetic findings in an extended family pedigree with sleepwalking. Neurol 2011;76(1):49–52.

32. Duncan L, Yilmaz Z, Gaspar H, et al. Significant locus and metabolic genetic correlations revealed in genome-wide association study of anorexia nervosa. Am J Psychiatry 2017;174(9):850–8.

33. Heidbreder A, Frauscher B, Mitterling T, et al. Not only sleepwalking but NREM parasomnia irrespective of the type is associated with HLA DQB1*0501. J Clin Sleep Med 2016;12(4):565–70.

34. Gaig C, Graus F, Compta Y, et al. Clinical manifestations of the anti-IgLON5 disease. Neurol 2017; 88(18):1736–43.

35. Gaig C, Iranzo A, Santamaria J, et al. The sleep disorder in anti-IgLON5 disease. Curr Neurol Neurosci Rep 2018;18(7):41.

36. Balint B, Antelmi E, Mencacci N, et al. Oculomotor apraxia and disrupted sleep with nocturnal ballistic bouts in ADCY5-related disease. Parkinsonism Relat Disord 2018;54:103–6.

37. Harris M, Grunstein RR. Treatments for somnambulism in adults: assessing the evidence. Sleep Med Rev 2009;13(4):295–7.

38. Kierlin L, Littner MR. Parasomnias and antidepressant therapy: a review of the literature. Front Psychiatry 2011;2:71.

39. Marwood L, Wise T, Perkins AM, et al. Meta-analyses of the neural mechanisms and predictors of response to psychotherapy in depression and anxiety. Neurosci Biobehav Rev 2018;95:61–72.

40. Tóth K, Csukly G, Sirok D, et al. Optimization of clonazepam therapy adjusted to patient's CYP3A status and NAT2 genotype. Int J Neuropsychopharmacol 2016;19(12):pyw083.

Sleep and Memory
The Promise of Precision Medicine

Patricia Carter, PhD, RN, CNS[a],*, Lichuan Ye, PhD, RN[b], Kathy Richards, PhD, RN[a],
Vani Vallabhaneni, MD[c]

KEYWORDS

- Sleep • Elderly • Mild cognitive impairment (MCI)
- Alzheimer's disease and related dementias (ADRD) • Precision sleep assessment
- Precision sleep treatment

KEY POINTS

- Up to 70% of people in early-stage dementia experience disturbed sleep. Frequent sleep disturbances include excessive nighttime awakenings, lower sleep efficiency, excessive daytime sleepiness, and increased daytime napping.
- Clinical and objective assessments indicate a high prevalence of comorbid sleep disorders in persons with mild cognitive impairment/Alzheimer's disease and related dementias (MCI/ADRD), notably chronic insomnia disorder, obstructive sleep apnea, circadian rhythm sleep-wake disorder, and restless legs syndrome.
- Due to the lack of accurate self-reports, challenges of performing polysomnography, or possible atypical manifestations, sleep disorders are commonly underdiagnosed and undertreated in older adults with MCI/ADRD.
- Nonpharmacologic therapies are recommended first-line therapies because they address psychosocial/environmental contributing factors for sleep disorders.
- Pharmacologic management in older adults with AD/ADRD can be a complex process. Drug-to-drug interactions and negative side effects must be carefully weighed when considering the addition of sleep medications.

INTRODUCTION

Sleep disturbances are frequent complaints in older adults with memory decline, defined as mild cognitive impairment (MCI)/Alzheimer's disease and related dementias (ADRD). Caregivers of persons with more severe manifestations of sleep and memory disturbance are affected too, and nighttime sleep disturbances are often cited by them as a major reason for nursing home admission of those they care for.

Data from polysomnography, actigraphy, direct observation, and clinical assessment provide objective evidence on a high prevalence of comorbid sleep disorders in persons with MCI/ADRD, notably chronic insomnia disorder, obstructive sleep apnea (OSA), circadian rhythm sleep-wake disorder, and restless legs syndrome (RLS). Unfortunately, the "secondary" nature of sleep disorders to memory decline, the questionable direction of causality, and diagnosis in persons with ADRD who may be unable to cognitively or verbally express their sleep symptoms may promote inadequate diagnosis and treatment.

Disclosure Statement: None of the authors associated with this publication have any conflicts of interest to disclose.
[a] School of Nursing, University of Texas at Austin, 1710 Red River Street, Austin, TX 78712, USA; [b] School of Nursing, Bouve College of Health Sciences, Northeastern University, 207c Robinson Hall, 360 Huntington Avenue, Boston, MA 02115, USA; [c] Texas A&M University, Sleep 360 Sleep Diagnostic Center, 10601 Pecan Park boulevard, Ste 203, Austin, TX 78750, USA
* Corresponding author.
E-mail address: pcarter@mail.nur.texas.edu

Sleep Med Clin 14 (2019) 371–378
https://doi.org/10.1016/j.jsmc.2019.05.001

Identification and management of other common comorbid medical disorders that affect sleep, such as major depression, chronic pain, nocturia, and delirium adds further complexity to treatment approaches for sleep disturbances in this population. Additional challenges to management of sleep disturbances in institutional settings (nursing home, assisted living, and acute care) include excessive noise, lack of light, inactivity, excessive time in bed, and interruptions to sleep for nighttime care practices. To achieve successful long-term outcomes, these multiple factors must be addressed using precision treatment approaches tailored to genetic, biomarker, phenotypic, and psychosocial characteristic of individuals with MCI/ADRD. We discuss here the significance of sleep disturbances in this population, contributing factors, assessment and diagnostic challenges, common sleep disorders and mechanisms, tailored behavioral and pharmacologic interventions, knowledge gaps, and provide ideas for future research.

SLEEP DISTURBANCES IN OLDER ADULTS WITH MEMORY DECLINE

As many as 70% of people in early-stage dementia experience disturbed sleep.[1] Frequent sleep disturbances reported in individuals with dementia include excessive nighttime awakenings, lower sleep efficiency, excessive daytime sleepiness, and increased napping during the day.[2] Such sleep disturbances can emerge in early-stage disease, and is associated with degree of the cognitive decline.[2] Various sleep disturbances may coexist. In a multicenter cross-sectional study on 431 Italian patients with MCI/ADRD, more than 60% of them reported comorbid sleep disturbances.[3] Electroencephalogram (EEG) changes have been reported in demented elderly. For example, there is a quantitative decrease in the rapid eye movement (REM) sleep specific to AD that has been proposed as a marker of AD.[4]

Sleep-wake rhythms can be severely impaired in elderly with MCI/ADRD. With the progression of dementia, the capacity to maintain both sleep and wakefulness are impaired, leading to circadian disturbances.[5] In a study of 171 individuals with dementia, Sullivan and Richards[6] found that 42% of patients with dementia had no discernible sleep-wake rhythm. Furthermore, institutionalized dementia patients' rhythms were so disturbed they could not maintain sleep or awake for a full hour within a 24-hour period.[5]

Sleep disturbances in individuals with dementia present a heavy burden for their caregivers, in particular spousal caregivers.[7] The cost of care for patients with dementia was estimated at $277 billion in 2018 and is expected to be more than $1.1 trillion by 2050.[8] A large portion of the cost arises from behavioral problems related to agitation, depression, and sleep disturbance. Frequent awakenings at night increase stress and burden in caregivers, which may prompt institutionalization of older adults.[7,9] Excessive noise, nighttime care practices, physical and social inactivity, and lack of bright light inherent in many institutional settings may further worsen sleep.[10] Therefore, identifying and managing sleep disturbances in dementia can be critically important to the well-being of both patients and caregivers.

FACTORS CONTRIBUTING TO SLEEP DISTURBANCES IN OLDER ADULTS WITH MEMORY DECLINE

The etiology of sleep disturbance in elderly with memory decline is multifactorial, including contributing factors such as cognitive impairment, environment, behavior, treatments, and comorbidities, among others. **Box 1** summarizes the factors that contribute to sleep disturbances in this population.

Sleep and Cognition: a Bidirectional Relationship

Mounting evidence suggests a bidirectional link between sleep disturbance and cognitive decline.[11,12] Recent mechanistic investigations have focused on the bidirectional relationship between sleep and cognition, with a strong interest in how sleep disturbances lead to cognitive decline.[13] For example, signature sleep abnormalities appear before clinical onset of AD, and sleep deprivation facilitates accumulation of amyloid-β, which may potentially trigger early cognitive decline and conversion to AD.[13] Although sleep disturbances might contribute to cognitive decline through pathways such as amyloid-β accumulation, neuro-inflammation, and alterations in specific neurotransmitters, the mechanisms are still poorly understood and might be modified by individual factors such as sex, APOE ε4 gene status, depression, and medication.[14] Although more research is needed to understand this bidirectional relationship, the available evidence suggests that sleep is an important modifiable target for developing strategies to treat memory decline or reduce dementia risks.[15]

Age-Related Changes

Although aging itself cannot explain poor sleep in older adults with memory decline, age-related changes such as lower sleep efficiency, longer sleep latency, and advanced sleep phase

Box 1
Factors that contribute to sleep disturbances in older adults with memory decline

Cognitive Function

- Cognitive impairment
- Alzheimer's disease or other types of dementia

Age-related Changes

- Changes in sleep architecture
- Advanced sleep phase
- Weakening of circadian entertainment
- Visual impairment

Environmental Factors

- Daytime limited exposure to bright light
- Nighttime environmental noise, light, and unpleasant temperature
- Room sharing
- Nocturnal care activities and facility routines for those in long-term care

Behavioral Factors

- Reduced daytime physical activity
- Social disengagement
- Excessive daytime napping

Primary Sleep Disorders

- Insomnia
- Sleep-related breathing disorders, particularly obstructive sleep apnea
- Sleep-related movement disorders, particularly restless legs syndrome

Medical and Psychiatric Comorbidities

- Incontinence and nocturia
- Symptoms such as pain and dyspnea
- Depression and other psychiatric problems
- Delirium
- Side effects of medications

contribute to greater sleep disturbance.[16] Weakening of circadian entrainment and visual impairment in older adults can contribute to sleep-wake rhythm abnormalities leading to greater sleep complaints.[17]

Environmental Factors

Sleep in older adults with memory decline can be interrupted by environmental factors such as excessive nocturnal noise and light exposure, low daytime light exposure, uncomfortable room temperature, and nocturnal care practices. Limited exposure to bright light during the day can significantly contribute to circadian deregulation.[18] Higher levels of agitation have been identified to be associated with lack of daytime bright light exposure and high levels of nocturnal light exposure in institutionalized patients with AD, which emphasizes the need for normal circadian light patterns.[19]

Behavioral Factors

Older adults with memory decline tend to be physically inactive, spend extended time in bed, and are less engaged in social activities during the day. Studies in nursing home residents suggest that reduced daytime physical activities and social disengagement can significantly contribute to circadian rhythm abnormalities resulting in excessive daytime sleepiness and disturbed nighttime sleep.[20–22] Excessive daytime napping may lead to decreased nocturnal sleep and alter the sleep-wake cycle.[5,20]

Primary Sleep Disorders

Sleep disorders are common in older adults with memory decline, but may be underdiagnosed and undertreated. In this population, sleep disorders are primarily represented by insomnia, sleep-related breathing disorders, particularly OSA, sleep-related movement disorder, particularly RLS, and circadian rhythm sleep-wake disorders. OSA causes intermittent hypoxia and sleep fragmentation and affects at least 20% of people older than 65 years.[23] It is estimated that up to 70% to 80% of older adults with AD/ADRD may have OSA,[22,24] and percent of time spent in apnea or hypopnea is positively associated with the severity of MCI/ADRD.[25] OSA can impact brain structure and function, and accumulating epidemiologic and mechanistic evidence supports that OSA is a risk factor for cognitive impairment and dementia[23,26] and treatment may slow cognitive decline.

Symptoms of cognitive dysfunction are common in persons with RLS.[27] RLS risk factors and behaviors are prevalent in persons with MCI/ADRD[21] and RLS is associated with nighttime agitation and wandering.[28,29] In a study comparing 16 patients with RLS with 15 age-matched and gender-matched healthy adults (47–72 years of age), patients with RLS compared with controls showed significant (P<.05) and sizable (20%–40%) deficits on 2 of 3 prefrontal cortical functioning tests.[27] In another study, conducted by Richards and colleagues, sleep was measured by 2 nights of in-home, attended polysomnography in 59 older adults with MCI/ADRD whose caregivers reported nighttime agitation. Nighttime agitation was measured over

3 additional nights by direct observation. Two experts independently and via consensus identified RLS using polysomnography, behavioral observations, sleep history from informants, and medical history data. Total sleep time in participants was 5.6 hours (SD 1.8 hours). Mean periodic limb movement index was 15.29, and a high percentage (49%) had moderate to severe OSA. RLS was present in 24% of participants. Severe cognitive impairment, low apnea-hypopnea index, and RLS were associated with nighttime agitation ($R^2 = 0.35$, $P<.001$).[29]

Medical and Psychiatric Comorbidities

Sleep complaints in older adults are often secondary to other comorbidities.[16] Elderly adults commonly experience multiple chronic medical conditions (eg, congestive health failure with nocturnal respiratory distress, chronic obstructive pulmonary disease, gastroesophageal reflux, chronic pain, and nocturia) that can directly interrupt their sleep. Psychiatric disorders are common, as suggested that approximately 50% of patients with AD may have symptoms of depression.[30] Defined as an acute disorder of attention and cognition, delirium is common, serious, and often fatal among older patients.[31] Delirium is characterized by disrupted a sleep-wake cycle, and disruption of sleep-wake cycle may also predispose individuals to develop delirium.[31,32] A wide range of medications used in the management of medical and psychiatric disorders can further contribute to sleep disturbances or impaired daytime alertness.[33] It is important to evaluate the use of both prescription and over-the-counter medications, as well as social drugs, such as caffeine, nicotine, and alcohol when evaluating sleep disturbances in elderly persons with MCI/ADRD.

CHALLENGES TO ASSESSING SLEEP DISTURBANCES IN OLDER ADULTS WITH MEMORY DECLINE
Sleep History

A personalized assessment of sleep and circadian disturbances should include a global geriatric approach, but be individually tailored. Because older adults with memory decline may not be aware of sleep problems or cannot recall symptoms accurately, it is essential to interview both patients and caregivers.[34] In addition to clinical features typically queried during a sleep assessment (eg, timing and regularity of sleep, naps during the day, symptoms for primary sleep disorders), clinicians should specifically ask about sundowning, sleep attacks, hallucinations, and nighttime wandering.[34] Clinical query should

consider comorbid medical and psychiatric conditions and contributing factors, such as pain, nocturnal respiratory distress, nocturia, depression, medication use, physical and social activity, and noise and light exposure.[34,35]

Sleep Scales

Commonly used sleep scales, such as the Epworth Sleepiness Scale (ESS)[36] and Pittsburgh Sleep Quality Index (PSQI),[37] have not been validated for use in individuals with memory decline, and their typical interpretive cutoffs may not be applicable to this population. Dementia-specific scales, such as the Sleep Disorders Inventory,[38] may be helpful to assess symptoms of sleep disturbances and sleep disorders in this population. A discrepancy between subjective and objective sleep disturbances reported in older adults with ADRD calls for more reliable objective evaluation.[39]

Polysomnogram

Polysomnogram (PSG) remains the "gold standard" for sleep assessment, and is required if a sleep disorder such as sleep apnea or Periodic Limb Movement Disorder is suspected. However, PSG can be difficult to obtain in cognitively impaired individuals because they may remove sensors and may not follow instructions. A caregiver should stay with the patient to assist with PSG, if possible, to minimize the confusion caused by an unfamiliar environment and numerous sensors.[34]

Actigraphy

Actigraphy can be a feasible alternative to PSG for objective measurement of sleep in nonlaboratory settings.[40] The standard practice committee of the American Academy of Sleep Medicine recommends actigraphy and sleep diaries to be routinely used to assess for sleep disturbances and circadian rhythm disorders in dementia.[41] In general, wrist and ankle actigraphy are well-tolerated in all but the most severely agitated older adults. It should be noted that actigraphy may not reliably distinguish sleep and wakefulness in individuals with Parkinson disease due to tremor or if there is limb movement disorder. Another disadvantage is that actigraphy is usually not reimbursed by insurers.[3]

Need for Tailored, Personalized Diagnostic Approaches for Sleep Disorders in Mild Cognitive Impairment/Alzheimer's Disease and Related Disorders

Due to the lack of accurate self-reports on sleep problems, challenges of performing polysomnography, or possible atypical manifestations, sleep disorders are commonly underdiagnosed and undertreated in older adults with MCI/ADRD. Current guidelines to screen and diagnose sleep disorders may not be applicable. There is a critical need to establish tailored screening and diagnostic tools for sleep disorders in this vulnerable population. Regarding REM sleep behavior disorder for instance, the Mayo sleep questionnaire bed-partner/informant version has been validated to screen for this disorder in older adults with dementia.[42]

One common sleep disorder that demonstrates the need for modification of its diagnostic approach is RLS. Given the sensory nature of RLS, current diagnostic standards emphasize self-report of symptoms, thus is unsuitable for persons with memory decline. Furthermore, RLS may be expressed only by nocturnal agitation in elderly with dementia, which may add to the difficulty identifying RLS in these patients.[29] Richards and colleagues[43] developed and validated an objective RLS diagnostic tool for use in dementia, the Behavioral Indicators Test–Restless Legs (BIT-RL). Consisting of a 20-minute observation for 8 behavioral indicators and an assessment for the 6 clinical indicators collected from chart review and caregiver interviews, the BIT-RL has demonstrated good diagnostic accuracy for RLS. This work in RLS is an exemplar for establishing diagnostic criteria of other sleep disorders in older adults with memory decline.

TREATMENT RECOMMENDATIONS

Nonpharmacologic therapies are recommended first-line therapies because they address psychosocial/environmental contributing factors for sleep disorders while avoiding drug side effects and drug-to-drug interactions.[11,44] Cognitive behavioral therapy, sleep hygiene, stimulus control, and sleep restriction have robust evidence to support their effectiveness in older adults. In addition to treating the sleep disturbance, common nonpharmacologic therapies are also indicated for frequent comorbid conditions. For example, regular physical exercise (sleep hygiene) is a strategy for insomnia because it may promote relaxation and raise core body temperature, which could help in initiating and maintaining sleep. Further, exercise has many additional benefits for older adults. In a 4-group randomized trial, Richards and colleagues[22] found that strength training and walking in combination with increased social activity significantly increased total sleep time, sleep efficiency, and non-REM sleep (measured by polysomnography) compared with a control group in 165 older adults with AD/ADRD. Exercise is also

indicated as an approach to lower blood pressure,[45] improve physical function,[46,47] improve cognitive functioning in the elderly,[48] and significantly lowers the apnea-hypopnea index in older adults with OSA and AD/ADRD.[24] Other lifestyle modifications (eg, weight loss) have the potential to reduce the severity of OSA as well as improve diabetic control. Manipulation of the environment to include bright light exposure is supported as a promising strategy for managing insomnia in the elderly with dementia.[49]

Although selection and administration of pharmacologic therapies routinely consider individual patient conditions, behavioral therapies may be the ones in greatest need for tailoring for individuals with MCI/ADRD. For example, cognitive behavioral therapy for insomnia (CBT-I) requires the individual to be able to engage in the education and practice elements of the therapy. In the case of moderate to severe memory impairment, the individual may not be able to learn and remember the information that the therapist provides. Recent work is beginning to explore ways to tailor broadly accepted behavioral approaches for common sleep disorders. Cassidy-Eagle and colleagues[50] found positive results in an MCI population with insomnia by modifying traditional CBT-I to decrease the amount of content covered, slowing the pace of delivery and increasing repetition of presented material, and providing regular reminders. An additional modification that could be useful for persons with moderate to severe MCI/ADRD would be to include a family member or caregiver in the therapy sessions with the patient to learn and help to apply the principles for improved sleep.

Continuous positive airway pressure (CPAP) therapy is another area in which a tailored approach to education and support can increase compliance with therapy. One approach that has shown promise is the inclusion of a supportive other (spouse, adult child, or friend) to remind and encourage routine use of CPAP therapy for those with MCI.[51,52] This could be extended further to include active participation of caregiver for application and maintenance of the CPAP device in persons with advanced AD/ADRD. In a prospective study using a tailored CPAP adherence intervention in older adults with MCI and OSA, adherence to CPAP defined as $\geq$ 4 hours of CPAP use over 1 year (n = 29), compared with a nonadherent control group (n = 25), resulted in approximately 55% adherence, and significant improvements in psychomotor/cognitive processing speed, after adjustment for baseline differences in age, race, and marital status.[51]

Institutional settings in which older persons with MCI/ADRD may live (eg, nursing homes, assisted living) or may be receiving episodic treatment (acute care, rehabilitation facilities) can also contribute to or exacerbate sleep disorders. Special considerations are required when providing care for older adults in these environments. A regular sleep-wake schedule, adequate lighting (eg, bright light in day and dim light at night), and minimization of noise and nighttime care disruptions have been shown to reduce delirium and to promote overall sleep quality.[44] Health care providers of persons with MCI/ADRD and sleep disturbances should work in collaboration with the patient and their families to identify outcome goals for improved sleep. Once these goals are established, specific treatment approaches can be discussed to arrive at a precision solution for each patient and family.

Pharmacologic management in older adults with AD/ADRD can be a complex process. Drug-to-drug interactions and negative side effects must be carefully weighed when considering the addition of sleep medications. For example, Z-drugs, melatonin receptor agonists, orexin receptor antagonists, and antidepressants are frequently prescribed for insomnia. However, older adults commonly experience significant side effects (dizziness, cardiac arrhythmias, delirium).[53] Specialty organizations have recognized the risks associated with pharmacologic management of sleep disorders in older adults and have issued clinical practice guidelines and clinical recommendations for treatment of sleep disorders in adults.[54] In addition, the Beers Criteria of the American Geriatrics Society (2015) have indicated that benzodiazepines and diphenhydramine should be avoided in older adults.[55]

SUMMARY AND FUTURE DIRECTIONS

Sleep disturbances are common in older adults with AD/ADRD, appear early in the course of memory decline, and severely affect the quality of life of patients, families, and caregivers. Further, growing evidence suggests that sleep disturbances may accelerate the trajectory of cognitive and functional decline, and neurodegeneration. Further research is needed to develop evidence-based precision medicine approaches to successfully prevent and treat sleep disturbances in older adults with memory decline. Importantly, future research also should determine the effect of treating sleep disturbances on cognitive decline, neurodegeneration, and other outcomes important to patients, families, and caregivers.

REFERENCES

1. Rongve A, Boeve BF, Aarsland D. Frequency and correlates of caregiver-reported sleep disturbances in a sample of persons with early dementia. J Am Geriatr Soc 2010;58(3):480–6.
2. Cole CS, Richards KC. Sleep in persons with dementia: increasing quality of life by managing sleep disorders. J Gerontol Nurs 2006;32(3):48–53.
3. Guarnieri B, Adorni F, Musicco M, et al. Prevalence of sleep disturbances in mild cognitive impairment and dementing disorders: a multicenter Italian clinical cross-sectional study on 431 patients. Dement Geriatr Cogn Disord 2012;33(1):50–8.
4. Petit D, Gagnon JF, Fantini ML, et al. Sleep and quantitative EEG in neurodegenerative disorders. J Psychosom Res 2004;56(5):487–96.
5. Pat-Horenczyk R, Klauber MR, Shochat T, et al. Hourly profiles of sleep and wakefulness in severely versus mild-moderately demented nursing home patients. Aging (Milano) 1998;10(4):308–15.
6. Sullivan SC, Richards KC. Predictors of circadian sleep-wake rhythm maintenance in elders with dementia. Aging Ment Health 2004;8(2):143–52.
7. Etters L, Goodall D, Harrison BE. Caregiver burden among dementia patient caregivers: a review of the literature. J Am Acad Nurse Pract 2008;20(8):423–8.
8. Alzheimer's Association. Alzheimer's disease facts and figures. Alzhimers Dement 2018;14(3):367–429.
9. Gaugler JE, Duval S, Anderson KA, et al. Predicting nursing home admission in the U.S: a meta-analysis. BMC Geriatr 2007;7:13.
10. Ye L, Richards KC. Sleep and long-term care. Sleep Med Clin 2018;13:117–25.
11. Guarnieri B, Sorbi S. Sleep and cognitive decline: a strong bidirectional relationship. It is time for specific recommendations on routine assessment and the management of sleep disorders in patients with mild cognitive impairment and dementia. Eur Neurol 2015;74(1–2):43–8.
12. Villa C, Ferini-Strambi L, Combi R. The synergistic relationship between Alzheimer's disease and sleep disorders: an update. J Alzheimers Dis 2015;46(3):571–80.
13. Mander BA, Winer JR, Jagust WJ, et al. Sleep: a novel mechanistic pathway, biomarker, and treatment target in the pathology of Alzheimer's disease? Trends Neurosci 2016;39(8):552–66.
14. Yaffe K, Falvey CM, Hoang T. Connections between sleep and cognition in older adults. Lancet Neurol 2014;13(10):1017–28.
15. Wennberg AMV, Wu MN, Rosenberg PB, et al. Sleep disturbance, cognitive decline, and dementia: a review. Semin Neurol 2017;37(4):395–406.
16. Foley D, Ancoli-Israel S, Britz P, et al. Sleep disturbances and chronic disease in older adults: results

of the 2003 National Sleep Foundation Sleep in America Survey. J Psychosom Res 2004;56(5): 497–502.

17. Zizi F, Jean-Louis G, Magai C, et al. Sleep complaints and visual impairment among older Americans: a community-based study. J Gerontol A Biol Sci Med Sci 2002;57(10):M691–4.

18. Shochat T, Martin J, Marler M, et al. Illumination levels in nursing home patients: effects on sleep and activity rhythms. J Sleep Res 2000;9(4):373–9.

19. Martin JL, Marler M, Shochat T, et al. Circadian rhythms of agitation in institutionalized patients with Alzheimer's disease. Chronobiol Int 2000;17(3):405–18.

20. Martin JL, Webber AP, Alam T, et al. Daytime sleeping, sleep disturbance, and circadian rhythms in the nursing home. Am J Geriatr Psychiatry 2006; 14(2):121–9.

21. Richards KC, Beck C, O'Sullivan PS, et al. Effect of individualized social activity on sleep in nursing home residents with dementia. J Am Geriatr Soc 2005;53(9):1510–7.

22. Richards KC, Lambert C, Beck CK, et al. Strength training, walking, and social activity improve sleep in nursing home and assisted living residents: randomized controlled trial. J Am Geriatr Soc 2011; 59(2):214–23.

23. Gosselin N, Baril AA, Osorio RS, et al. Obstructive sleep apnea and the risk of cognitive decline in older adults. Am J Respir Crit Care Med 2019; 199(2):142–8.

24. Herrick JE, Bliwise DL, Puri S, et al. Strength training and light physical activity reduces the apnea-hypopnea index in institutionalized older adults. J Am Med Dir Assoc 2014;15(11):844–6.

25. Ancoli-Israel S, Klauber MR, Butters N, et al. Dementia in institutionalized elderly: relation to sleep apnea. J Am Geriatr Soc 1991;39(3):258–63.

26. Baril AA, Carrier J, Lafrenière A, et al. Biomarkers of dementia in obstructive sleep apnea. Sleep Med Rev 2018;42:139–48.

27. Pearson VE, Allen RP, Dean T, et al. Cognitive deficits associated with restless legs syndrome (RLS). Sleep Med 2006;7:25–30.

28. Richards K, Shue VM, Beck CK, et al. Restless legs syndrome risk factors, behaviors, and diagnoses in persons with early to moderate dementia and sleep disturbance. Behav Sleep Med 2010;8(1):48–61.

29. Rose KM, Beck C, Tsai PF, et al. Sleep disturbances and nocturnal agitation behaviors in older adults with dementia. Sleep 2011;34(6):779–86.

30. Migliorelli R, Tesón A, Sabe L, et al. Prevalence and correlates of dysthymia and major depression among patients with Alzheimer's disease. Am J Psychiatry 1995;152(1):37–44.

31. Oh ES, Fong TG, Hshieh TT, et al. Delirium in older persons: advances in diagnosis and treatment. JAMA 2017;318(12):1161–74.

32. Fitzgerald JM, Adamis D, Trzepacz PT, et al. Delirium: a disturbance of circadian integrity? Med Hypotheses 2013;81(4):568–76.

33. Foral P, Knezevich J, Dewan N, et al. Medication-induced sleep disturbances. Consult Pharm 2011; 26(6):414–25.

34. Ooms S, Ju YE. Treatment of sleep disorders in dementia. Curr Treat Options Neurol 2016;18(9):40.

35. Urrestarazu E, Iriarte J. Clinical management of sleep disturbances in Alzheimer's disease: current and emerging strategies. Nat Sci Sleep 2016;8: 21–33.

36. Johns MW. A new method for measuring daytime sleepiness: the Epworth sleepiness scale. Sleep 1991;14(6):540–5.

37. Buysse DJ, Reynolds CF 3rd, Monk TH, et al. The Pittsburgh Sleep Quality Index: a new instrument for psychiatric practice and research. Psychiatry Res 1989;28(2):193–213.

38. Tractenberg RE, Singer CM, Cummings JL, et al. The Sleep Disorders Inventory: an instrument for studies of sleep disturbance in persons with Alzheimer's disease. J Sleep Res 2003;12(4):331–7.

39. Most EI, Aboudan S, Scheltens P, et al. Discrepancy between subjective and objective sleep disturbances in early- and moderate-stage Alzheimer disease. Am J Geriatr Psychiatry 2012;20(6): 460–7.

40. Van de Water AT, Holmes A, Hurley DA. Objective measurements of sleep for non-laboratory settings as alternatives to polysomnography—a systematic review. J Sleep Res 2011;20(1 Pt 2):183–200.

41. Morgenthaler T, Alessi C, Friedman L, et al. Practice parameters for the use of actigraphy in the assessment of sleep and sleep disorders: an update for 2007. Sleep 2007;30(4):519–29.

42. Boeve BF, Molano JR, Ferman TJ, et al. Validation of the Mayo Sleep Questionnaire to screen for REM sleep behavior disorder in an aging and dementia cohort. Sleep Med 2011;12(5):445–53.

43. Richards KC, Bost JE, Rogers VE, et al. Diagnostic accuracy of behavioral, activity, ferritin, and clinical indicators of restless legs syndrome. Sleep 2015; 38(3):371–80.

44. Praharaj SK, Gupta R, Gaur. Clinical practice guideline on management of sleep disorders in the elderly. Indian J Psychiatry 2018;60(suppl3): S383–96.

45. Bonardi JMT, Lima LG, Campos GO, et al. Effect of different types of exercise on sleep quality of elderly subjects. Sleep Med 2016;25:122–9.

46. Lorenz RA, Gooneratne N, Cole CS. Exercise and social activity improve everyday function in long-term care residents. Am J Geriatr Psychiatry 2012; 20(6):468–76.

47. Cole CS, Richards KC, Beck C, et al. Relationships among disordered sleep and cognitive and

functional status in nursing home residents. Res Gerontol Nurs 2009;2(3):183–91.

48. Northey JM, Cherbuin N, Pumpa KL, et al. Exercise interventions for cognitive function in adults older than 50: a systematic review with meta-analysis. Br J Sports Med 2018;52(3):154–60.

49. Sekiguchi H, Iritani S, Fujita K. Bright light therapy for sleep disturbance in dementia is most effective for mild to moderate Alzheimer's type dementia: a case series. Psychogeriatrics 2017;17: 275–81.

50. Cassidy-Eagle E, Siebern A, Until L, et al. Neuropsychological functioning in older adults with mild cognitive impairment and insomnia randomized to CBT-I or control group. Clin Gerontol 2018;41(2): 136–44.

51. Richards KC, Gooneratne N, Dicicco B, et al. CPAP adherence may slow 1-year cognitive decline in older adults with mild cognitive impairment and apnea. J Am Geriatr Soc 2019;67(3):558–64.

52. Sawyer AM, Gooneratne NS, Marcus CL, et al. A systematic review of CPAP adherence across age groups: clinical and empiric insights for developing CPAP adherence interventions. Sleep Med Rev 2011;15(6):343–6.

53. Mets MA, de Vries JM, de Senerpoint Dormis LM, et al. Next-day effects of ramelteron (8mg), Zopiclone (7.5mg), and placebo on highway driving performance, memory functioning, psychomotor performance, and mood in healthy adult subjects. Sleep 2011;34(10):1327–34.

54. Sateia MJ, Buysse DJ, Krystal AD, et al. Clinical practice guideline for the pharmacologic treatment of chronic insomnia in adults: an American Academy of Sleep Medicine clinical practice guideline. J Clin Sleep Med 2017;13(2):307–49.

55. American Geriatrics Society 2012 Beers Criteria Update Expert Panel. American Geriatrics Society updated Beers Criteria for potentially inappropriate medication use in older adults. J Am Geriatr Soc 2015;63(11):2227–46.

Further Development of P4 Approach to Obstructive Sleep Apnea

Allan I. Pack, MBChB, PhD

KEYWORDS

- Obstructive sleep apnea • Personalized medicine • Cardiovascular disease • Cluster analyses

KEY POINTS

- There are distinct clinical subtypes of obstructive sleep apnea (OSA): (a) patients who have insomnia as their primary complaint; (b) patients who are asymptomatic; (c) patients with excessive sleepiness.
- The benefit of CPAP therapy for OSA varies between these clinical subtypes.
- The increased cardiovascular risk as a result of OSA only occurs in the excessively sleepy subtype.

INTRODUCTION

The fundamental concept that underlies the concept of personalized medicine is that all individuals with the same disorder are not the same. There are various factors that contribute to the unique aspects of individual patients. These include the following: genetics (both common and rare variants), microbiome, epigenetic modifications, and environment. The environment can have direct effects and also may modify the microbiome and methylation patterns on DNA. Hypermethylation at specific sites on DNA leads to alteration in corresponding gene expression.

If we accept that these differences between patients with the same disease exist, then there are likely to be different pathways to disease, different consequences, and different responses to therapy. The approach is not to assume that one knows the differences that exist, but rather to use unbiased approaches to identify the differences. Differences are assessed in multiple dimensions. These include the following: clinical features, for example, symptoms; consequences of disease; physiologic differences, for example, features of sleep study; molecular profiles using all omics approaches (metabolomics, transcriptomics, and proteomics); imaging differences; and other deep phenotyping strategies. These assessments are combined with new analytical strategies such as machine learning, as well as unsupervised clustering analysis to identify subgroups. This requires study and characterization of large numbers of patients. In time, new classifications of disease will develop and be used clinically. In this brief review, I discuss some current approaches to developing personalized approaches to obstructive sleep apnea (OSA).

P4 MEDICINE

One particular "variety" of personalized medicine is P4 medicine.[1,2] There are previous reviews on this topic applying it to OSA.[3,4] This concept was developed by Dr. Leroy Hood.[1,2] The 4 Ps are: predictive, preventative, personalize, and participatory.

The fundamental concept is that, as we move forward, we will try to maintain health by predicting illness and seeking to prevent it. When disease occurs, diagnosis and treatment will be personalized. The fourth P—participatory—indicates that techniques should be deployed to engage the individual in recognizing their own disease at an early point and be involved in their own disease management. The development of mobile devices

Disclosure: Funding for this work was provided in part by NIH grant P01 HL094307.
Translational Research Laboratories, Center for Sleep and Circadian Neurobiology, University of Pennsylvania Perelman School of Medicine, Suite 2100, 125 South 31st Street, Philadelphia, PA 19104-3403, USA
E-mail address: pack@mail.med.upenn.edu

Sleep Med Clin 14 (2019) 379–389
https://doi.org/10.1016/j.jsmc.2019.05.004
1556-407X/19/

and involvement of companies such as Fitbit, Apple, and Google are intended to facilitate a consumer-based, rather than a physician-driven, health care approach. This will require not only technological development, validation of the technology, but also considerable education of the public. We now discuss some of the different efforts to develop a personalized approach to OSA.

DISEASE PATHOGENESIS

With respect to pathogenesis, the fundamental concept is that development of obstructive sleep apnea depends on structural and physiologic risk factors. Structural risk factors include alteration in soft tissues[5,6] and craniofacial dimensions.[7–9] Both size of soft tissues[10] and craniofacial dimensions[11] are heritable.

Physiologic risk factors have been defined by Owen and colleagues.[12] They are the following: airway collapsibility; loop gain, a measure of ventilatory control stability; arousal threshold; and upper airway muscle responsiveness to negative intraluminal pressure. These variables can be determined by quite complex studies during sleep.[12] There is some indication that second-line therapies for OSA could be based on the different physiologic risk factors.[13,14] However, these studies have, of necessity, given their complex nature, been done in very small samples of patients. Recently there have been efforts to extract these variables from routine sleep studies, albeit based on a model of ventilatory drive.[15] There has been some validation of this new approach, but we are still a long way from these concepts being applied clinically. We need to show that the data obtained are stable from night to night and obtain data on a large enough sample to allow machine-learning/clustering approaches to be applied.

Structural risk factors are also important. The relative role of soft tissues and craniofacial dimensions vary by ethnic group.[16,17] If one compares patients with the same level of severity of OSA who are white and those who are Chinese,[17] white people are more obese and have increased tongue size, whereas Chinese have more craniofacial restriction.[17] Chinese are more sensitive to increased body mass index (BMI) such that the slope of the line showing the relationship between severity of OSA and BMI is steeper in Chinese. This presumably is the result of their craniofacial restriction. As a result, OSA in Asians is a somewhat different disease. In Taiwan, for example, there are many patients in their 30s who are not obese but have severe OSA.[18] Given the increasing rates of obesity in China,[19] there could

be an epidemic of OSA in China. China has a limited number of sleep physicians, sleep technologists, and so forth, to cope with this epidemic.

PHYSIOLOGIC SUBTYPES

One dimension to consider for evaluation of differences is the nature of the physiologic disturbances during sleep. This has been addressed by Zinchuk and colleagues,[20] who considered all of the variables that are extracted routinely from polysomnography (PSG). When they applied cluster analyses they found 7 subtypes (**Table 1**). Two of the subtypes had what would be considered mild OSA, 2 moderate, and 3 severe (see **Table 1**). These data were obtained from a cohort in the VA system. The investigators were able to assess the rate of subsequent cardiovascular (CV) events in these patients and compare the rates of CV events in each of the 7 groups in those who used continuous positive airway pressure (CPAP) treatment and those who did not. They found that CPAP altered the rate of CV events in only 2 of the 7 groups. The result was somewhat surprising because the groups comprised 1 with mild OSA but significant periodic limb movements, and 1 with severe OSA, hypopneas, and hypoxia.

This approach is clearly interesting and could be useful in determining which patients are at risk for CV disease. Although Zinchuk and colleagues[20] used standard metrics from the PSG, there are now a large number of novel measures that can be obtained from the PSG by new analytical strategies. Some examples of these measures include the following: (a) total oxygen desaturation area[21,22]; (b) assessment of arousal intensity[23] (c) odds ratio product (ORP), a continuous measure of sleep depth[24]; (d) ORP 9, that is, ORP 9 seconds after an arousal that indicates the speed of returning to sleep[25]; (e) heart rate response to arousal, a heritable trait[26,27]; (f) cardiopulmonary coupling during sleep, another measure of sleep depth,[28] and (g) respiratory event duration.[29] Heart rate response to arousal is a physiologic measure of interest as twin studies demonstrate that it is heritable, and that responses within individuals are stable across nights but variable between individuals.[26,27] Respiratory event duration has also received attention because there are both long and short events, which can occur on the same night in the same individual.[29] The frequency of short events are associated with objective measures of daytime sleepiness; longer events are associated with hypertension.[29] Family-based studies show that the average duration of respiratory events is heritable.[30] It is conceivable that analysis of PSG data using this

Table 1
The 7 clusters identified by Zinchuk et al[20] based on analysis of data obtained from routine polysomnograms

Description of and labels for the polysomnographic clusters based on distinguishing features

Cluster (n)	Cluster label	Median AHI (events/hour)	Conventional OSA severity	
A (533)	Mild	4		
			None/mild	
B (119)	PLMS	10		⟶ CPAP reduces CV events
C (186)	NREM and poor sleep	19		
			Moderate	
D (168)	REM and hypoxia	19		
E (75)	Hypopnoea and hypoxia	44		⟶ CPAP reduces CV events
F (42)	Arousal and poor sleep	68	Severe	
G (124)	Combined severe	84		

In only 2 clusters was there evidence that CPAP treatment of OSA reduces cardiovascular events.
From Zinchuk AV, Jeon S, Koo BB, Yan X, Bravata DM, Qin L, Selim BJ, Strohl KP, Redeker NS, Concato J, Yaggi HK. Polysomnographic phenotypes and their cardiovascular implications in obstructive sleep apnoea. Thorax 2018;73(5):472–80; with permission.

increased number of variables will reveal even more informative physiologic subtypes.

CLINICAL SUBTYPES

Another dimension to consider is symptoms. We conducted a study to evaluate the differences in symptoms in patients with OSA with colleagues in Iceland using the Icelandic Sleep Apnea Cohort.[31] The Icelandic clinical team administered detailed questionnaires to all new patients being evaluated for CPAP therapy. Unsupervised clustering revealed that there were 3 clinical subtypes: (a) individuals in whom the main complaint was difficulty initiating or maintaining sleep, that is, insomnia; (b) a group who were relatively asymptomatic and wake up feeling refreshed; and (c) a group who were excessively sleepy[31] (**Box 1**). These differences were not explained by the severity of OSA or BMI, which were essentially identical in all 3 groups (**Table 2**).

A commentary on this article correctly pointed out that it would be important to show that these subgroups were generalizable and not simply related to referral patterns in Iceland.[32] We therefore sought to replicate these findings in other cohorts. First, with our Korean colleagues, we replicated that the subtypes existed in the Korean Genomic Cohort.[33,34] In this population-based cohort the prevalence of the excessively sleepy group was lower than in the Icelandic clinical cohort. This is in line with the findings that OSA is common in population-based studies but the symptom burden is low.[35]

We also replicated the subtypes in the Sleep Apnea Global Interdisciplinary Consortium (SAGIC) (for details, see Magalang and colleagues[36,37]). This consortium is made up of leading sleep centers around the world (**Fig. 1**) and its goal is to develop novel approaches to diagnosis and treatment of OSA. Each site administers the same questionnaires to all patients recruited and collects craniofacial photographs[38] and intraoral pictures.[39] These photographs are analyzed at the University of Sydney and the University of group with moderate sleepiness and a group with a predominance of upper airway symptoms They had high rates of snoring, witnessed apneas and waking suddenly unable to breathe.[40] We therefore, believe that fundamentally there are different cluster subtypes based on symptoms The 3 major subtypes—insomnia, asymptomatic and excessively sleepy—are found in all studies.

The existence of these subtypes raises the question as to whether the outcomes after initiation of therapy vary by subtype. In the Icelandic Sleep Apnea Cohort, changes in symptoms were evaluated after 2 years of CPAP therapy.[41] In the insomnia group, there was a smaller proportion of subjects still complaining of insomnia symptoms after 2 years, although many individuals continued to have these complaints even with effective CPAP therapy (**Fig. 2**). This suggests that for some individuals with OSA and insomnia, the insomnia is caused by the OSA (waking up as a result of respiratory events), whereas for others insomnia is caused by other mechanisms. Even though this group had at baseline, on average a normal Epworth Sleepiness Score (ESS), there was a small but significant improvement with therapy (see **Fig. 2**). The asymptomatic group, which at baseline did not report falling asleep inappropriately during the day or while driving, not surprisingly, had the lowest improvements in symptoms with therapy (**Fig. 3**). However in this group, there was a significant improvement in the proportion of patients experiencing excessive sleepiness and a small but significant change in ESS (see **Fig. 3**). Not surprisingly, the largest changes in symptoms occurred in the excessively sleepy group (**Fig. 4**). Large improvements were shown in the proportion of patients complaining of falling asleep inappropriately and feeling drowsy while driving (see **Fig. 4**). No other group showed this difference. This group showed a large change in ESS (see **Fig. 4**).

Pennsylvania, respectively. Saliva or blood are obtained for DNA analysis. All questionnaire data are put into REDCap, which is housed at Ohio State University. All sleep studies are uploaded to a server at the University of Sydney, Australia. When we assessed clusters based on questionnaire data across all sites, the same 3 subtypes were identified,[40] as described in Iceland,[31] and 2 additional clusters. The other 2 clusters were a

Table 2
The gender, age, body mass index, and severity of obstructive sleep apnea (average apnea-hypopnea index) in the 3 clusters identified in the Icelandic Sleep Apnea Cohort

	Total Cohort	Cluster 1	Cluster 2	Cluster 3	
Number of Subjects	823	252 (30.6%)	209 (25.4%)	362 (44.0%)	*P* Value
Male (%)	80.9	83.3	77.5	81.2	.280[a]
Age (y), μ ± SD	54.5 ± 10.6	53.1 ± 10.7	55.1 ± 10.5	55.1 ± 10.5	.102[b]
BMI (kg/m²), μ ± SD	33.5 ± 5.7	33.8 ± 5.8	33.1 ± 5.7	33.4 ± 5.7	.355[b]
AHI (events/h), μ ± SD	44.8 ± 20.7	44.5 ± 20.6	46.1 ± 19.8	44.5 ± 21.3	.421[b]

Cluster 1 is the insomnia group, cluster 2 is relatively asymptomatic, and cluster 3 is the excessively sleepy group. Cluster differences are not driven by BMI or AHI.
Abbreviations: AHI, apnea-hypopnea index; BMI, body mass index.
[a] Difference in the distribution of gender among 3 clusters was examined by Pearson's chi-square test.
[b] Differences in age, BMI, and AHI among 3 clusters were examined by Kruskal-Wallis equality-of-population rank tests

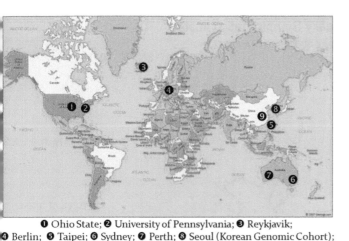

Fig. 1. International sites for Sleep Apnea Global Interdisciplinary Consortium (SAGIC).

❶ Ohio State; ❷ University of Pennsylvania; ❸ Reykjavik;
❹ Berlin; ❺ Taipei; ❻ Sydney; ❼ Perth; ❽ Seoul (Korean Genomic Cohort);
❾ Beijing/Shanghai

Although there are differences in symptomatic changes with CPAP in the 3 groups, whether other outcomes, in particular CV events, are different between the groups has not been well established. To address this, we studied data from the Sleep Heart Health Study (SHHS). This large study, based on community (not clinical) samples, was designed to assess the association between OSA and different aspects of CV disease.[42–53] Demographic data, questionnaire data, sleep study

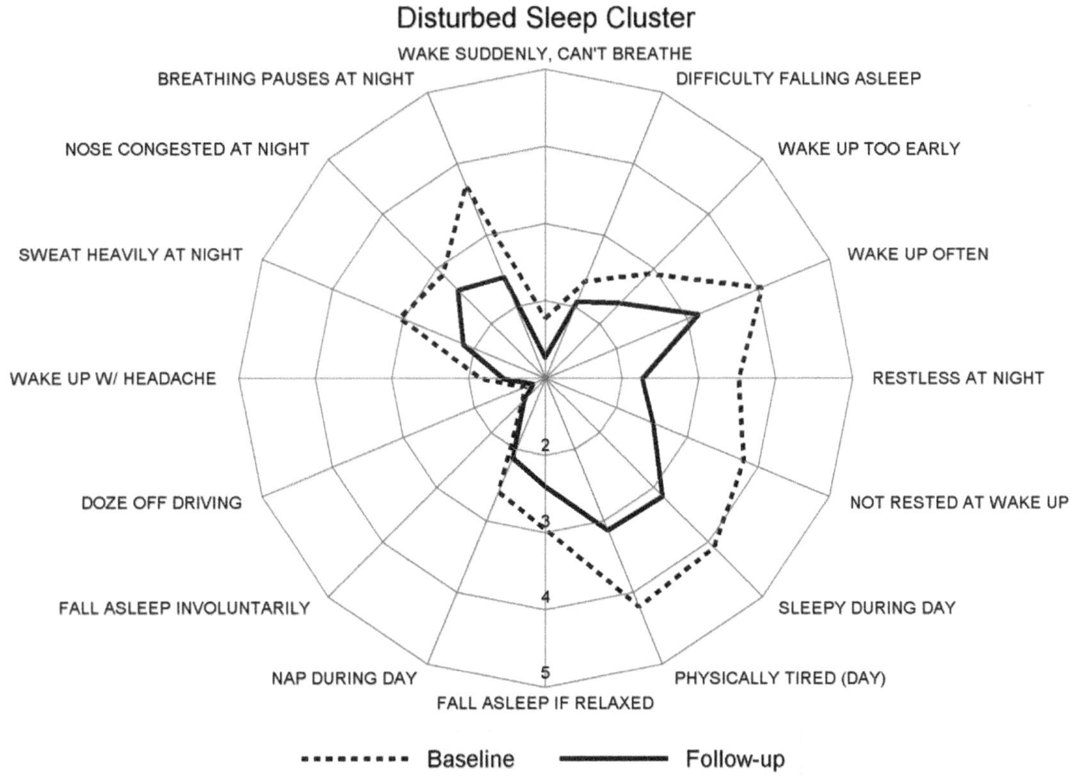

Disturbed Sleep Cluster

WAKE SUDDENLY, CAN'T BREATHE
BREATHING PAUSES AT NIGHT
DIFFICULTY FALLING ASLEEP
NOSE CONGESTED AT NIGHT
WAKE UP TOO EARLY
SWEAT HEAVILY AT NIGHT
WAKE UP OFTEN
WAKE UP W/ HEADACHE
RESTLESS AT NIGHT
DOZE OFF DRIVING
NOT RESTED AT WAKE UP
FALL ASLEEP INVOLUNTARILY
SLEEPY DURING DAY
NAP DURING DAY
PHYSICALLY TIRED (DAY)
FALL ASLEEP IF RELAXED

·········· Baseline   ———— Follow-up

Fig. 2. Radar plot showing number of subjects endorsing a particular symptom before (*dashed line*) and after (*solid line*) therapy. In this insomnia group, there is improvement in the number of patients restless at night, waking up often, as well as complaints of being sleepy during the day. The group did not report falling asleep involuntarily or dozing off while driving. Change in Epworth Sleepiness Score = −2.06 (*P*<.001). (*From* Pien GW, Ye L, Keenan BT, Maislin G, Bjornsdottir E, Arnardottir ES, Benediktsdottir B, Gislason T, Pack AI. Changing faces of obstructive sleep apnea: treatment effects by cluster designation in the Icelandic Sleep Apnea Cohort. Sleep 2018;41(3); with permission.)

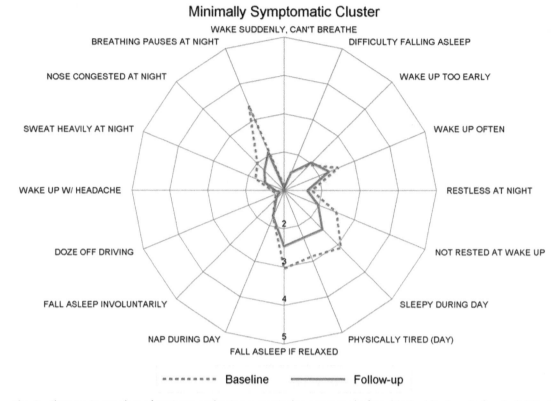

Fig. 3. Changes in number of patients endorsing a particular symptom before (*dashed line*) and after (*solid line*) treatment in asymptomatic group. The changes in this group are, as anticipated, much smaller than in other groups. Even in this group, however, there is a change in the number of subjects indicating being sleepy or physically tired during the day. Change in Epworth Sleepiness Score = −1.33 (*P*<.001). (*From* Pien GW, Ye L, Keenan BT, Maislin G, Bjornsdottir E, Arnardottir ES, Benediktsdottir B, Gislason T, Pack AI. Changing faces of obstructive sleep apnea: treatment effects by cluster designation in the Icelandic Sleep Apnea Cohort. Sleep 2018;41(3); with permission.)

results, and information about incident CV events were obtained from the National Sleep Research Resource.[54,55] Although the questionnaires used in the SHHS are not identical to those used in Icelandic Sleep Apnea Cohort or SAGIC, there was sufficient information to do unsupervised clustering. We found the 3 major symptomatic subtypes of OSA in individuals with an apnea-hypopnea index greater than 15 events/h. The optimal cluster solution, however, had 4 subgroups, with the fourth group being characterized by moderate sleepiness.[56]

The rate of incident cardiac events was assessed over the median 11.8 years of follow-up. We examined the rate of events related to the following: coronary artery disease, heart failure, and finally all CV events. Survival analyses (**Fig. 5**) showed that there was an increased rate of all 3 types of cardiac events in the excessively sleepy group compared with the other 3 subgroups and to controls without OSA. To assess more definitively the risk of CV events in the different subtypes of OSA, we carried out a

case-control analysis for each of the 4 subtypes. In adjusted analyses, we found that only the excessively sleepy group, compared with controls without OSA, had a significantly increased rate of events related to coronary heart disease (left panel, **Fig. 6**), heart failure (middle panel, **Fig. 6**), and all CV events (right panel, **Fig. 6**). Thus, the major risk of CV events in subjects with OSA was in the excessively sleepy group.

This is not the first study to suggest the role of excessive sleepiness. The presence of sleepiness increases the association between OSA and hypertension.[57,58] A recent study of OSA in patients with myocardial infarction also demonstrated the importance of sleepiness.[59] In this study individuals who had a myocardial infarction had sleep studies to identify the presence of OSA. Subjects with untreated OSA, who have an ESS greater than 10, have an increased rate of reinfarction and major CV events than those who have normal ESS[59] (**Fig. 7**).

The basis of this effect of sleepiness is currently unknown. It is conceivable that it could be the

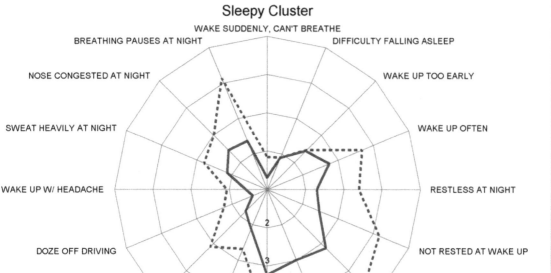

Fig. 4. Radar plot showing change in number of patients in excessively sleeping subgroup endorsing particular symptoms before (*dashed line*) to after 2 years of CPAP therapy (*solid line*). There are large symptomatic improvements in this group and a large change in Epworth Sleepiness Score. This is the only group who report falling asleep involuntarily and dosing off while driving. This improves with therapy. There is a large, significant reduction in Epworth Sleepiness Score. Change in Epworth Sleepiness Score = −5.31 (P<.001). (*From* Pien GW, Ye L, Keenan BT, Maislin G, Bjornsdottir E, Arnardottir ES, Benediktsdottir B, Gislason T, Pack AI. Changing faces of obstructive sleep apnea: treatment effects by cluster designation in the Icelandic Sleep Apnea Cohort. Sleep 2018;41(3); with permission.)

result of different physiologic derangements during sleep that result not only in sleepiness but also increased risk for CV events. It could also be that the differences are genetic or epigenetic.

Altered inflammatory response to sleep-disordered breathing is a possibility,[60] as are differences in choline levels.[61] Future studies need to address the basis of this difference.

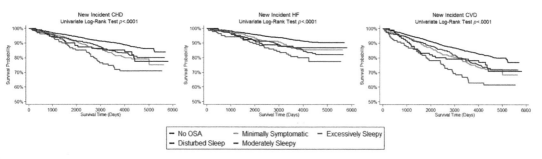

Fig. 5. Survival curves showing data for new incident coronary heart disease (CHD) (*left panel*), heart failure (HF) (*middle panel*), and all cardiovascular disease (CVD) (*right panel*). Data are shown for the 4 clinical subtypes and for individuals with an apnea-hypopnea index less than 5 events/h (no OSA). For each outcome there are more incident events in the excessively sleepy group. Covariates in adjusted analyses: age, sex, body mass index, type 2 diabetes, hypertension, high-density lipoprotein, total cholesterol, triglycerides, alcohol use, and smoking status.

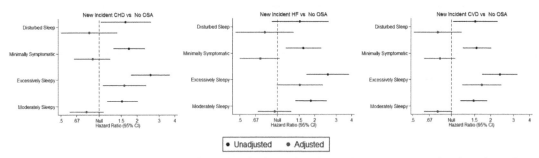

Fig. 6. Hazard ratios with 95% CI in unadjusted and adjusted analyses. The covariates used in the adjusted analyses are described below. The figure shows the hazard ratio compared with controls without OSA for each of the 4 symptomatic groups in the Sleep Heart Health Study. The data shown are for incident coronary heart disease (CHD) (*left panel*), heart failure (HF) (*middle panel*), and incident of all cardiovascular disease (CVD) (*right panel*). After adjustment, the increased risk for each of the 3 cardiovascular outcomes occurs only in the excessively sleepy group. Covariates in adjusted analyses: age, sex, body mass index, type 2 diabetes, hypertension, high density lipoprotein, total cholesterol, triglycerides, alcohol use, and smoking status.

Whatever the basis for the difference, this result has important implications (see editorial on this study[62]). In particular, it may explain, at least in part, the negative results of the recent large randomized trial (SAVE) of CV events in patients with moderate-to-severe OSA.[63] This trial excluded patients with marked excessive sleepiness (ESS >15) given concerns that randomizing this group to no therapy might result in an increased rate of motor vehicle crashes. However

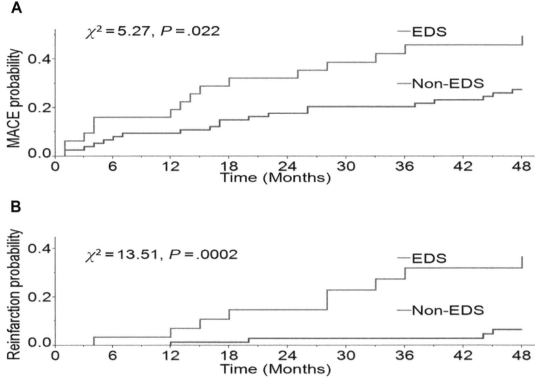

Fig. 7. Rates of reinfarction (panel B) and major cardiovascular events (panel A) in individuals with OSA who are excessively sleepy (EDS) and nonexcessively sleepy (non-EDS). Excessively sleepy was defined based on a threshold of the Epworth Sleepiness Score. The P values refer to the significance of differences between groups. MACE is major adverse cardiac events; EDS defined as Epworth Sleepiness Score ≥11. (*From* Xie J, Sert Kuniyoshi FH, Covassin N, Singh P, Gami AS, Chahal CAA, Somers VK. Excessive daytime sleepiness independently predicts increased cardiovascular risk after myocardial infarction. Journal of the American Heart Association 2018;7(2); with permission.)

excluding this group suggests that the individuals with the greatest risk for CV disease were actually excluded. Future studies in this area need to find ways to conduct studies on the effect of CPAP on CV events that include individuals with marked excessive sleepiness. One approach, used by us in studies of effects of CPAP treatment of OSA on lipid levels, might involve propensity score matching, comparing the outcomes of individuals who are very adherent to CPAP to those who do not use it.[64]

PARTICIPATORY CARE—THE FINAL P

The final P in the P4 approach is participatory. As a field, we are in a terrific position to implement this approach. Modern CPAP machines provide a wealth of data remotely. These data can be obtained by providers and given to the patients themselves. Providing CPAP adherence data to patients with OSA enhances CPAP compliance.[65]

Moving forward, there are substantial new developments in the area of mobile devices[66] and specialized mattresses[67] that will provide further opportunities for patients to engage in their own care.

SUMMARY

We are currently at an early point in developing personalized approaches to diagnosis and management of OSA. There are, however, already indications that we will change the way we approach patients with this common disorder. There are major opportunities for further developing a P4 approach to obstructive sleep apnea.

REFERENCES

1. Cesario A, Auffray C, Russo P, et al. P4 medicine needs P4 education. Curr Pharm Des 2014;20(38): 6071–2.
2. Sagner M, McNeil A, Puska P, et al. The P4 health spectrum - a predictive, preventive, personalized and participatory continuum for promoting healthspan. Prog Cardiovasc Dis 2017;59(5):506–21.
3. Pack AI. Application of personalized, predictive, preventative, and participatory (P4) medicine to obstructive sleep apnea. A roadmap for improving care? Ann Am Thorac Soc 2016;13(9):1456–67.
4. Lim DC, Sutherland K, Cistulli PA, et al. P4 medicine approach to obstructive sleep apnoea. Respirology 2017;22(5):849–60.
5. Schwab RJ, Gupta KB, Gefter WB, et al. Upper airway and soft tissue anatomy in normal subjects and patients with sleep-disordered breathing. Significance of the lateral pharyngeal walls. Am J Respir Crit Care Med 1995;152(5 Pt 1):1673–89.
6. Kim AM, Keenan BT, Jackson N, et al. Tongue fat and its relationship to obstructive sleep apnea. Sleep 2014;37(10):1639–48.
7. Sakamoto Y, Yanamoto S, Rokutanda S, et al. Predictors of obstructive sleep apnoea-hypopnea severity and oral appliance therapy efficacy by using lateral cephalometric analysis. J Oral Rehabil 2016;43(9):649–55.
8. Chi L, Comyn FL, Mitra N, et al. Identification of craniofacial risk factors for obstructive sleep apnoea using three-dimensional MRI. Eur Respir J 2011; 38(2):348–58.
9. Neelapu BC, Kharbanda OP, Sardana HK, et al. Craniofacial and upper airway morphology in adult obstructive sleep apnea patients: a systematic review and meta-analysis of cephalometric studies. Sleep Med Rev 2017;31:79–90.
10. Schwab RJ, Pasirstein M, Kaplan L, et al. Family aggregation of upper airway soft tissue structures in normal subjects and patients with sleep apnea. Am J Respir Crit Care Med 2006;173(4):453–63.
11. Chi L, Comyn FL, Keenan BT, et al. Heritability of craniofacial structures in normal subjects and patients with sleep apnea. Sleep 2014;37(10):1689–98.
12. Owens RL, Edwards BA, Eckert DJ, et al. An integrative model of physiological traits can be used to predict obstructive sleep apnea and response to non positive airway pressure therapy. Sleep 2015;38(6):961–70.
13. Sands SA, Edwards BA, Terrill PI, et al. Identifying obstructive sleep apnoea patients responsive to supplemental oxygen therapy. Eur Respir J 2018; 52(3) [pii:1800674].
14. Landry SA, Joosten SA, Sands SA, et al. Response to a combination of oxygen and a hypnotic as treatment for obstructive sleep apnoea is predicted by a patient's therapeutic CPAP requirement. Respirology 2017;22(6):1219–24.
15. Sands SA, Edwards BA, Terrill PI, et al. Phenotyping pharyngeal pathophysiology using polysomnography in patients with obstructive sleep apnea. Am J Respir Crit Care Med 2018;197(9):1187–97.
16. Sutherland K, Lee RWW, Chan TO, et al. Craniofacial phenotyping in Chinese and caucasian patients with sleep apnea: influence of ethnicity and sex. J Clin Sleep Med 2018;14(7):1143–51.
17. Lee RW, Vasudavan S, Hui DS, et al. Differences in craniofacial structures and obesity in Caucasian and Chinese patients with obstructive sleep apnea. Sleep 2010;33(8):1075–80.
18. Sutherland K, Keenan BT, Bittencourt L, et al. For the SAGIC investigators. A global comparison of anatomic risk factors and their relationship to obstructive sleep apnea severity in clinical samples. J Clin Sleep Med 2019;15(4):629–39.
19. Nie P, Ding L, Sousa-Poza A. Decomposing adult obesity trends in China (1991-2011). Econ Hum Biol 2019. https://doi.org/10.1016/j.ehb.2019.02.001.

20. Zinchuk AV, Jeon S, Koo BB, et al. Polysomnographic phenotypes and their cardiovascular implications in obstructive sleep apnoea. Thorax 2018; 73(5):472–80.

21. Azarbarzin A, Sands SA, Stone KL, et al. The hypoxic burden of sleep apnoea predicts cardiovascular disease-related mortality: the osteoporotic fractures in men study and the sleep heart health study. Eur Heart J 2019;40(14):1149–57.

22. Kulkas A, Duce B, Leppanen T, et al. Gender differences in severity of desaturation events following hypopnea and obstructive apnea events in adults during sleep. Physiol Meas 2017;38(8):1490–502.

23. Amatoury J, Azarbarzin A, Younes M, et al. Arousal intensity is a distinct pathophysiological trait in obstructive sleep apnea. Sleep 2016;39(12): 2091–100.

24. Younes M, Ostrowski M, Soiferman M, et al. Odds ratio product of sleep EEG as a continuous measure of sleep state. Sleep 2015;38(4):641–54.

25. Younes M, Hanly PJ. Immediate postarousal sleep dynamics: an important determinant of sleep stability in obstructive sleep apnea. J Appl Physiol (1985) 2016;120(7):801–8.

26. Azarbarzin A, Ostrowski M, Younes M, et al. Arousal responses during overnight polysomnography and their reproducibility in healthy young adults. Sleep 2015;38(8):1313–21.

27. Gao X, Azarbarzin A, Keenan BT, et al. Heritability of heart rate response to arousals in twins. Sleep 2017; 40(6). https://doi.org/10.1093/sleep/zsx055.

28. Thomas RJ, Mietus JE, Peng CK, et al. Relationship between delta power and the electrocardiogram-derived cardiopulmonary spectrogram: possible implications for assessing the effectiveness of sleep. Sleep Med 2014;15(1):125–31.

29. Koch H, Schneider LD, Finn LA, et al. Breathing disturbances without hypoxia are associated with objective sleepiness in sleep apnea. Sleep 2017; 40(11). https://doi.org/10.1093/sleep/zsx152.

30. Liang J, Cade BE, Wang H, et al. Comparison of heritability estimation and linkage analysis for multiple traits using principal component analyses. Genet Epidemiol 2016;40(3):222–32.

31. Ye L, Pien GW, Ratcliffe SJ, et al. The different clinical faces of obstructive sleep apnoea: a cluster analysis. Eur Respir J 2014;44(6):1600–7.

32. Ryan CM, Kendzerska T, Wilton K, et al. The different clinical faces of obstructive sleep apnea (OSA), OSA in older adults as a distinctly different physiological phenotype, and the impact of OSA on cardiovascular events after coronary artery bypass surgery. Am J Respir Crit Care Med 2015;192(9): 1127–9.

33. Kim J, Keenan BT, Lim DC, et al. Symptom-based subgroups of Koreans with obstructive sleep apnea. J Clin Sleep Med 2018;14(3):437–43.

34. Kim NH, Seo JA, Cho H, et al. Risk of the development of diabetes and cardiovascular disease in metabolically healthy obese people: the Korean Genome and Epidemiology Study. Medicine (Baltimore) 2016;95(15):e3384.

35. Arnardottir ES, Bjornsdottir E, Olafsdottir KA, et al. Obstructive sleep apnoea in the general population highly prevalent but minimal symptoms. Eur Respir J 2016;47(1):194–202.

36. Magalang UJ, Johns JN, Wood KA, et al. Home sleep apnea testing: comparison of manual and automated scoring across international sleep centers. Sleep Breath 2019;23(1):25–31.

37. Magalang UJ, Arnardottir ES, Chen NH, et al. Agreement in the scoring of respiratory events among international sleep centers for home sleep testing. J Clin Sleep Med 2016;12(1):71–7.

38. Sutherland K, Schwab RJ, Maislin G, et al. Facial phenotyping by quantitative photography reflects craniofacial morphology measured on magnetic resonance imaging in Icelandic sleep apnea patients. Sleep 2014;37(5):959–68.

39. Schwab RJ, Leinwand SE, Bearn CB, et al. Digital morphometrics: a new upper airway phenotyping paradigm in OSA. Chest 2017;152(2):330–42.

40. Keenan BT, Kim J, Singh B, et al. Recognizable clinical subtypes of obstructive sleep apnea across international sleep centers: a cluster analysis. Sleep 2018;41(3). https://doi.org/10.1093/sleep/zsx214.

41. Pien GW, Ye L, Keenan BT, et al. Changing faces of obstructive sleep apnea: treatment effects by cluster designation in the Icelandic Sleep Apnea Cohort. Sleep 2018;41(3). https://doi.org/10.1093/sleep/zsx201.

42. Ogilvie RP, Lakshminarayan K, Iber C, et al. Joint effects of OSA and self-reported sleepiness on incident CHD and stroke. Sleep Med 2018;44:32–7.

43. Aurora RN, Crainiceanu C, Gottlieb DJ, et al. Obstructive sleep apnea during REM sleep and cardiovascular disease. Am J Respir Crit Care Med 2018;197(5):653–60.

44. Tung P, Levitzky YS, Wang R, et al. Obstructive and central sleep apnea and the risk of incident atrial fibrillation in a community cohort of men and women. J Am Heart Assoc 2017;6(7) [pii:e004500].

45. Roca GQ, Redline S, Claggett B, et al. Sex-specific association of sleep apnea severity with subclinical myocardial injury, ventricular hypertrophy, and heart failure risk in a community-dwelling cohort: the Atherosclerosis Risk in Communities-Sleep Heart Health Study. Circulation 2015;132(14):1329–37.

46. Gottlieb DJ, Yenokyan G, Newman AB, et al. Prospective study of obstructive sleep apnea and incident coronary heart disease and heart failure: the sleep heart health study. Circulation 2010;122(4) 352–60.

47. Redline S, Yenokyan G, Gottlieb DJ, et al. Obstructive sleep apnea-hypopnea and incident stroke

the sleep heart health study. Am J Respir Crit Care Med 2010;182(2):269–77.

48. Punjabi NM, Caffo BS, Goodwin JL, et al. Sleep-disordered breathing and mortality: a prospective cohort study. PLoS Med 2009;6(8):e1000132.

49. O'Connor GT, Caffo B, Newman AB, et al. Prospective study of sleep-disordered breathing and hypertension: the sleep heart health study. Am J Respir Crit Care Med 2009;179(12):1159–64.

50. Punjabi NM, Newman AB, Young TB, et al. Sleep-disordered breathing and cardiovascular disease: an outcome-based definition of hypopneas. Am J Respir Crit Care Med 2008;177(10):1150–5.

51. Newman AB, Nieto FJ, Guidry U, et al. Relation of sleep-disordered breathing to cardiovascular disease risk factors: the sleep heart health study. Am J Epidemiol 2001;154(1):50–9.

52. Shahar E, Whitney CW, Redline S, et al. Sleep-disordered breathing and cardiovascular disease: cross-sectional results of the sleep heart health study. Am J Respir Crit Care Med 2001;163(1):19–25.

53. Nieto FJ, Young TB, Lind BK, et al. Association of sleep-disordered breathing, sleep apnea, and hypertension in a large community-based study. Sleep heart health study. JAMA 2000;283(14):1829–36.

54. Dean DA 2nd, Goldberger AL, Mueller R, et al. Scaling up scientific discovery in sleep medicine: the national sleep research resource. Sleep 2016; 39(5):1151–64.

55. Zhang GQ, Cui L, Mueller R, et al. The national sleep research resource: towards a sleep data commons. J Am Med Inform Assoc 2018;25(10):1351–8.

56. Mazzotti DR, Keenan BT, Lim DC, et al. Symptom subtypes of obstructive sleep apnea predict incidence of cardiovascular outcomes. Am J Respir Crit Care Med 2019. https://doi.org/10.1164/rccm.201808-1509OC.

57. Kapur VK, Resnick HE, Gottlieb DJ. Sleep disordered breathing and hypertension: does self-reported sleepiness modify the association? Sleep 2008;31(8):1127–32.

58. Lindberg E, Berne C, Franklin KA, et al. Snoring and daytime sleepiness as risk factors for hypertension and diabetes in women–a population-based study. Respir Med 2007;101(6):1283–90.

59. Xie J, Sert Kuniyoshi FH, Covassin N, et al. Excessive daytime sleepiness independently predicts increased cardiovascular risk after myocardial infarction. J Am Heart Assoc 2018;7(2) [pii: e007221].

60. Prasad B, Steffen AD, Van Dongen HPA, et al. Determinants of sleepiness in obstructive sleep apnea. Sleep 2018. https://doi.org/10.1093/sleep/zsx199.

61. Pak VM, Dai F, Keenan BT, et al. Lower plasma choline levels are associated with sleepiness symptoms. Sleep Med 2018;44:89–96.

62. Zinchuk A, Yaggi HK. Sleep apnea heterogeneity, phenotypes, and cardiovascular risk: implications for trial design and precision sleep medicine. Am J Respir Crit Care Med 2019. https://doi.org/10.1164/rccm.201903-0545ED.

63. McEvoy RD, Antic NA, Heeley E, et al. CPAP for prevention of cardiovascular events in obstructive sleep apnea. N Engl J Med 2016;375(10):919–31.

64. Keenan BT, Maislin G, Sunwoo BY, et al. Obstructive sleep apnoea treatment and fasting lipids: a comparative effectiveness study. Eur Respir J 2014;44(2):405–14.

65. Kuna ST, Shuttleworth D, Chi LQ, et al. Web-based access to positive airway pressure usage with or without an initial financial incentive improves treatment use in patients with obstructive sleep apnea. Sleep 2015;38(8):1229–36.

66. Bianchi MT. Sleep devices: wearables and nearables, informational and interventional, consumer and clinical. Metabolism 2018;84:99–108.

67. Tuominen J, Peltola K, Saaresranta T, et al. Sleep parameter assessment accuracy of a consumer home sleep monitoring ballistocardiograph Beddit Sleep Tracker: a validation study. J Clin Sleep Med 2019;15(3):483–7.

Precision Medicine for Obstructive Sleep Apnea

Matthew Light, MD*, Robert L. Owens, MD, Christopher N. Schmickl, MD, PhD, Atul Malhotra, MD

KEYWORDS

• Arousal threshold • Loop gain • Obstructive sleep apnea • OSA Treatment • Precision medicine

KEY POINTS

- The mechanisms underlying obstructive sleep apnea (OSA) are highly variable given that any single factor explains only a portion of the variance in OSA occurrence.
- The apnea-hypopnea index (AHI) is an imperfect metric of disease severity, because various complications are predicted by different sleep-disordered breathing variables, for example, 4% desaturation predicts hypertension, whereas 2% desaturation predicts insulin resistance. Similarly, arousal frequency predicts memory consolidation, and the duration of oxyhemoglobin saturation less than 90% predicts platelet aggregation. Thus, the optimal AHI definition may vary with the outcome of interest.
- Not all patients with OSA are at risk of the same complications. Cluster analyses and clinical trials suggest that some patients with OSA are at risk of cardiovascular complications, whereas others may be at risk of neurocognitive sequelae, and still others may remain asymptomatic.
- Although continuous positive airway pressure (CPAP) remains the treatment of choice for OSA, personalized medicine approaches are being used to optimize adherence to therapy. Examples include wearable technology with real-time patient feedback, which may help engage motivated patients and encourage CPAP use.
- Different interventions are now being tried to treat OSA based on endotypes (mechanisms) underlying the disease. Oxygen or acetazolamide may be effective for patients with unstable ventilatory control (high loop gain), whereas palatal surgery may be effective for patients with primarily an anatomic problem at the level of the velopharynx.

GENERAL CONSIDERATIONS

Obstructive sleep apnea (OSA) is a common condition with major neurocognitive and cardiovascular sequelae.[1] The disease is characterized by repetitive collapse of the pharyngeal airway during sleep yielding repetitive hypoxemia and hypercapnia with associated catecholamine surges. This breathing pattern leads to sleep fragmentation and autonomic changes that predispose to associated disease consequences.[2] Although commonly thought to be purely a result of upper airway crowding (frequently attributed to obesity), obstructive apneas do not occur during wakefulness.[3] In addition, there is considerable overlap in airway collapsibility (as measured by passive critical closing pressure or Pcrit technique) between patients with OSA and controls such that clearly other mechanisms are involved.[4] Recent studies have emphasized the variability in OSA

Disclosure Statement: The authors do not have any relationship with a commercial company that has direct financial interest in the subject matter or materials discussed in this article or with any company making a competing product. The authors did not receive any funding for this work.
Division of Pulmonary, Critical Care and Sleep Medicine, University of California San Diego, 9300 Campus Point Drive #7381, La Jolla, CA 92037-7381, USA
* Corresponding author.
E-mail address: mlight@ucsd.edu

Sleep Med Clin 14 (2019) 391–398
https://doi.org/10.1016/j.jsmc.2019.05.005
1556-407X/19/© 2019 Elsevier Inc. All rights reserved.

both from the standpoint of mechanisms underlying disease (ie, endotypes) as well as from sequelae of disease (ie, phenotypes).[5,6] As a result of this variability, OSA is being considered a disease amenable to precision medicine from the standpoint of diagnosis, treatment, as well as prognostication.[7]

PATHOGENESIS AND ENDOTYPES

Anatomic compromise at the level of the pharyngeal airway is necessary, although not always sufficient, for the development of OSA.[8,9] Based on imaging as well as assessment of mechanics, patients with OSA are at risk of pharyngeal collapse as compared with matched controls.[10] The patency of the pharyngeal airway is maintained during wakefulness ostensibly through protective pharyngeal reflexes that increase pharyngeal dilator muscle activity and prevent upper airway collapse.[11] As one example, the genioglossus muscle has phasic activity (bursts with each inspiration) and is state-dependent (has higher activity during wakefulness than during sleep) and has been extensively studied in this context.[12] The decrease in activity of the genioglossus muscle (and other upper airway dilators) at the onset of sleep may lead to pharyngeal collapse in those who are anatomically predisposed.[13]

Control of breathing may also be important in OSA pathogenesis.[14–16] Loop gain is an engineering term used to define the stability or instability in a feedback control system. A system with high loop gain is one which is prone to instability, whereas a system with low loop gain is intrinsically stable. A high loop gain system may develop oscillations with minor perturbations, whereas a system with low loop gain is one that will remain stable even with marked perturbations. Fluctuations in output from the respiratory central pattern generator in the brainstem lead to oscillations in activity of both the diaphragm and the upper airway dilator muscles. Thus, patients with high loop gain (and an anatomic predisposition) may develop upper airway collapse and obstruction when output to the upper airway dilator muscles is at its nadir.[17]

The ability to tolerate reductions in ventilation—the respiratory arousal threshold—is often variable between people and has also received recent attention.[18–20] Some patients have a low arousal threshold (wake up easily), whereas others have a high arousal threshold (sleep soundly).[21] Evidence suggests that most patients with OSA have some periods of stable breathing that occur spontaneously and are thought to result from activation of upper airway dilator muscles by endogenous stimuli (eg, CO_2, negative intrapharyngeal pressure).[22,23] In patients with a high arousal threshold, the accumulation of these respiratory stimuli can lead to activation of pharyngeal dilator muscles and thus periods of stable breathing. In contrast, patients with a low arousal threshold may have repetitive apneas. In this setting recurrent arousals from sleep reduce the period for sufficient accumulation of respiratory stimuli such that pharyngeal protective reflexes are not engaged.

Although the abovementioned factors are reasonably well established, recent emphasis has been placed on individual variability in each of these traits (endotypes). Some patients have primarily an anatomic problem predisposing them to pharyngeal collapse, whereas others have dysfunction in the upper airway dilator muscles, and still others have unstable ventilatory control (high loop gain) predisposing to pharyngeal collapse. It is not uncommon for patients to have multiple abnormalities that may be underlying OSA.[24,25]

Most of the concepts described earlier treat the upper airway as a collapsible tube with uniform collapsibility (ie, Starling resistor). One of the features of the Starling resistor is flow limitation such that increasing respiratory effort will not lead to increased flow. However, in practice a variety of flow patterns are observed across patients, which suggest that upper airway behavior is more complex.[26] Moreover, Azarbarzin and colleagues[27] have recently suggested that the different flow pattern "signatures" can be used to predict the variable sites of airway collapse. At least, in theory, 2 patients with the same collapsibility (as measured by passive Pcrit) might have very different anatomy and may respond differently to the same therapy aimed at improving anatomy, such as an oral appliance.

The personalized medicine approach to treating OSA involves recognition of this individual variability. Different interventions are available to influence each of these traits and may be effective strategies to treat OSA at least in select individuals and especially in those patients intolerant of continuous positive airway pressure (CPAP). For example, uvulopalatopharyngoplasty may be a useful strategy for patients who have OSA as a result of anatomic compromise at the level of the velopharynx.[28,29] Similarly, implantable hypoglossal nerve stimulators are effective in a subset of patients with OSA, although there are substantial barriers to this modality including cost, the need for multiple invasive procedures, and the inability to accurately predict responders.[30–32] On the other hand, surgical interventions may be neffective in patients who primarily have an issue with unstable ventilatory control.[33] Another example is the use of oxygen or acetazolamide, which are 2 strategies to lower loop gain and have been shown to be effective in a subset of patients with OSA.[34] Similarly, nonmyorelaxant hypnotic agents (eg, trazodone or eszopiclone) have been shown to increase the arousal threshold and may be useful in reducing sleep-disordered breathing events in select patients with a low arousal threshold predisposing to OSA.[35,36] In contrast, hypnotics may be ineffective or even deleterious in patients who have other underlying OSA mechanisms. Combination interventions have also been tried with some success to treat OSA in patients with multiple endotypes.[25]

DETERMINING THE OBSTRUCTIVE SLEEP APNEA ENDOTYPE

The challenge of determining the mechanisms underlying OSA has been the subject of extensive investigation.[37] Traditional assessment of the OSA endotype required multiple overnight experiments conducted by an MD or PhD to assess patients' physiology and to determine the magnitude of the variables (eg, pharyngeal collapsibility, loop gain, arousal threshold). However, recent emphasis has been placed on making these techniques more accessible to clinicians such that pathophysiologic traits could be estimated without the need for complex experiments. Several approaches have been used. First, Sands and colleagues[38] have recently used signal processing techniques to analyze standard polysomnography to make estimates of the various endotypes underlying OSA.[39] Orr and colleagues[40] have extended some of these findings to allow the assessment of some traits using home sleep testing. Further work will be required to validate these techniques and to determine their clinical utility. Second, Edwards and colleagues[20] have developed a regression equation to determine the arousal threshold using variables derived from standard polysomnography. For example, using the apnea-hypopnea index (AHI), the nadir saturation, and the presence of hypopneas and apneas, the investigators were able to define greater than 60% of the variance in the arousal threshold. Such efforts may allow the clinician to classify patients without the need for sophisticated physiologic testing that may be burdensome and limit willingness to participate in the diagnostic process. Third, technological innovations are allowing acquisition of data using wearable technologies or using blood biomarkers to help to draw conclusions. For example, technologies are being developed to assess sleep stages and oxygen levels in individuals, which may allow the assessment of pathophysiologic traits. Shin and colleagues have also reported in abstract form the ability to predict the arousal threshold using serum biomarkers such as high-sensitivity C-reactive protein and fasting blood glucose. Ongoing metabolomics research may further these efforts as well.[41] More work is required, but the realization that OSA is more than just an anatomic disease has opened the door to a personalized medicine approach to sleep apnea treatment.

OBSTRUCTIVE SLEEP APNEA PHENOTYPES

Although endotypes have been extensively studied, the variable OSA phenotypes have received less attention. Phenotypes have been described using various techniques. For example, Ye and colleagues[6] performed cluster analyses on large cohorts and found that patients with OSA have varying symptoms. Some have daytime sleepiness, others have difficulty sleeping at night, and there are those who remain relatively asymptomatic. These observations have been extended to other cohorts that have also demonstrated that symptoms change with CPAP treatment according to the original cluster.[6,42,43] Zinchuk and colleagues[44] also used cluster analysis and were able to risk stratify patients with OSA more effectively based on polysomnographic variables than with the AHI alone. The realization that not all patients with OSA are at risk of the same complications has several implications. First, further mechanistic research is imperative to determine why some patients with OSA get some complications, whereas others seem relatively protected. Secondly, with respect to clinical trials, a "one size fits all" strategy of trying to prevent a particular OSA consequence (eg, cardiovascular disease) by giving all patients with OSA nasal CPAP may be ineffective if only a subset is at risk. Finally, these findings also have clinical implications because interventions may be tailored to reduce the risk of a particular complication in a patient with a specific predisposition.

SUMMARY: WHY ENDOPHENOTYPES MATTER

There are several reasons why understanding OSA mechanisms on an individualized basis may facilitate a personalized medicine approach to therapy:

a. Endotype predicts phenotype. As stated, the mechanisms underlying OSA are highly variable as are the disease manifestations. In theory, OSA from a particular underlying

mechanism may have different disease consequences than OSA caused by a different mechanism. As one example, OSA in the elderly
seems to be more a function of upper airway
anatomy and less an issue with loop gain as
compared with younger patients with
OSA.[45–47] The authors and other investigators
have hypothesized that the mechanisms underlying OSA in the elderly may explain the lack of
observed complications in these patients in
some large epidemiologic cohorts.[48,49] On the
other hand, younger patients with OSA tend
to have higher loop gain, which may increase
risk of cardiovascular disease, as large, negative pleural pressure excursions can adversely
affect cardiac loading conditions and ventricular wall stress.

  b. Endotype determines response to therapy.
     Nasal CPAP therapy is highly efficacious but
     not always well tolerated. Stanchina and col-
     leagues[50] observed that patients with OSA
     with high loop gain might be at risk of devel-
     oping treatment-emergent central apneas on
     therapy (ie, complex OSA) and thus may not
     tolerate CPAP as well as other patients with
     OSA.[51] Such findings have implications for indi-
     vidual patient management, because patients
     likely to have an inadequate response to
     CPAP would ideally be identified *a priori* such
     that other interventions could be considered.
     Another example, which the authors and other
     investigators have recently observed, is that
     patients with unstable ventilatory control (high
     loop gain) are more likely to fail upper airway
     surgery with OSA as compared with matched
     individuals with low loop gain.[33,52] These find-
     ings may be helpful to stratify which patients
     are likely to benefit (or not) from a particular sur-
     gical intervention.
  c. Diseases associated with OSA may predispose
     based on specific endotypes. Several studies
     have suggested that patients with posttrau-
     matic stress disorder are at risk of OSA
     although the mechanisms are unclear.[53,54]
     Based on available data, the authors have
     speculated that such individuals may have a
     low arousal threshold and thus may be at risk
     of developing OSA on this basis. Similarly,
     certain patients with neuromuscular disease
     are known to be at risk of OSA, perhaps due
     to impairment in upper airway dilator muscle
     function.
  d. Endotype may define individualized interven-
     tional strategies. The use of oxygen and/or hyp-
     notics is likely to be beneficial for some patients
     with OSA but not for others, depending on un-
     derlying mechanisms.

Based on the conceptual framework discusse
earlier, the authors believe that OSA endophenc
types have essential implications for advancin
OSA management. They may soon be used i
the clinic to deliver a precision medicine-styl
approach to patient care (**Fig. 1**), and ultimatel
they may drive the future success of OSA clinica
trials such that efforts will focus on high-risk pa
tients who are most likely to benefit from a partic
ular intervention (**Fig. 2**).[55]

SUMMARY AND FUTURE DIRECTIONS

New insights into OSA have opened the door t
personalized medicine whereby individual patier
characteristics can help guide management. How
ever, many questions remain unanswered:

  a. How should endotype be best determined in th
     clinic and should these assessments chang
     management? Ultimately the answer to thi
     question will likely involve sophisticated ana
     lyses of physiologic signals (eg, from polysom
     nogram, home sleep testing, or wearabl
     technology) combined with plasma biomarkers
  b. Should patients with OSA known to be at risk c
     various disease complications be treated in a
     individualized manner, for example, should a
     otherwise healthy patient with OSA predicte
     to be at high risk of OSA-induced cardiovascu
     lar complications receive statin therapy an
     aggressive lifestyle modification? Such deci
     sions may be guided by underlying OSA mech
     anisms and by risk stratification using nove
     techniques.
  c. How should new biomarkers be best discov
     ered in the OSA field? Advances have bee
     made using exosomes, microRNAs and metab
     olomics/lipidomics that have allowed discover
     of new potential causal pathways to dis
     ease.[56,57] Recent insights into the microbiom
     have added the possibility that OSA affect
     gut bacteria, which in turn alter the associate
     metabolites important in the pathogenesis c
     atherosclerosis.[58]
  d. How can positive airway pressure (PAP) adher
     ence be best optimized using new technology
     Recent publications have shown potential ben
     efits to patient engagement and interactiv
     educational devices.[59,60] Our clinical experi
     ence suggests that ultimately different patient
     will respond to varying strategies, for example
     intensive support versus real-time patient feed
     back versus monetary incentives or othe
     approaches.[61,62]
  e. How will wearable technology affect OSA diag
     nosis   and   treatment   in   the   future

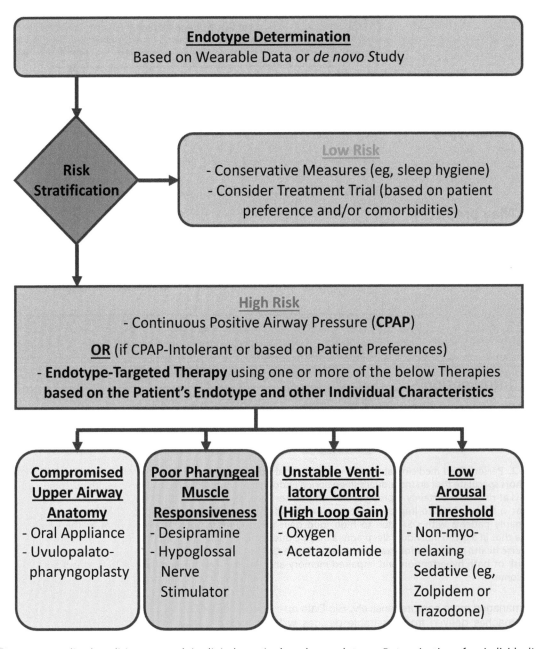

Fig. 1. Personalized medicine approach in clinical practice based on endotypes. Determination of an individual's endotype could be used for risk stratification to help decide *whether* (aggressive) treatment is indicated. In high-risk patients who are CPAP intolerant, this information could further be used to tailor therapy toward the individual's underlying sleep apnea causes. Note that in a given individual sleep apnea may potentially be due to multiple traits, thus requiring combination therapy; for example, a patient may have sleep apnea due to both high loop gain and low arousal threshold and may thus require both oxygen and a sedative in order to achieve stable breathing at night.

Technological advances may well allow OSA diagnosis and some sleep assessment to occur on an ongoing basis. Such data may be helpful diagnostically and may motivate behavioral changes such as improving sleep hygiene, and increasing PAP use. As the capability of wearable devices improve, the 3 pillars of health (diet, exercise, and sleep) could be

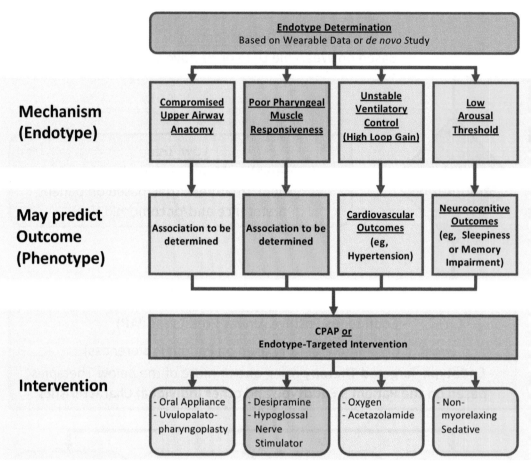

Fig. 2. Personalized medicine approach in clinical trial design based on endotypes. As discussed in the text, the authors speculate that an individual's sleep apnea endotype may predict which adverse health outcomes this person is at risk for; it certainly is predictive of which interventions other than CPAP may be efficacious. In this paradigm, a trial seeking to improve hypertension would maximize its power (ie, chance of success) by enrolling primarily patients with OSA due to high loop gain using CPAP (or potentially oxygen) as the intervention. Note that in a given individual sleep apnea may be due to more than one trait, thus increasing the risk of several adverse health outcomes; for example, a patient with OSA from high loop gain and low arousal threshold may be at risk of both hypertension and impaired memory and thus be a good candidate for trials focusing on either outcome.

managed more comprehensively. Big Data approaches derived from wearable devices will allow more robust conclusions over time.

OSA is an exciting field due to the tremendous progress that has been made in our understanding over recent years. The future looks bright because patients are yet to fully realize the benefits from fresh insights into sleep science and recent advancements in technology that are ongoing. OSA endophenotypes, an expanded array of OSA biomarkers, and a new wearable technology are 3 key elements that are currently leaping bench to bedside and are likely to have a significant impact on the substantial burden of disease-facing society.

REFERENCES

1. Jordan AS, McSharry DG, Malhotra A. Adult obstructive sleep apnoea. Lancet 2014;383(9918): 736–47.
2. Caples SM, Gami AS, Somers VK. Obstructive sleep apnea. Ann Intern Med 2005;142(3):187–97.
3. Welch K, Foster G, Ritter C, et al. A novel volumetric magnetic resonance imaging paradigm to study upper airway anatomy. Sleep 2002;25:532–42.
4. Gleadhill I, Schwartz A, Wise R, et al. Upper airway collabsibility in snorers and in patients with obstructive hypopnea and apnea. Am Rev Respir Dis 1991; 143:1300–3.
5. Eckert DJ, White DP, Jordan AS, et al. Defining phenotypic causes of obstructive sleep apnea.

Identification of novel therapeutic targets. Am J Respir Crit Care Med 2013;188(8):996–1004.

6. Ye L, Pien GW, Ratcliffe SJ, et al. The different clinical faces of obstructive sleep apnoea: a cluster analysis. Eur Respir J 2014;44(6):1600–7.

7. Pack AI. Application of personalized, predictive, preventative, and participatory (P4) medicine to obstructive sleep apnea. A roadmap for improving care? Ann Am Thorac Soc 2016;13(9):1456–67.

8. Haponik E, Smith P, Bohlman M, et al. Computerized tomography in obstructive sleep apnea: correlation of airway size with physiology during sleep and wakefulness. Am Rev Respir Dis 1983;127:221–6.

9. Schwab R, Pasirstein M, Pierson R, et al. Identification of upper airway anatomic risk factors for obstructive sleep apnea with volumetric magnetic resonance imaging. Am J Respir Crit Care Med 2003;168:522–30.

10. Isono S, Remmers JE, Tanaka A, et al. Anatomy of pharynx in patients with obstructive sleep apnea and in normal subjects. J Appl Physiol (1985) 1997;82(4):1319–26.

11. Mezzanotte WS, Tangel DJ, White DP. Waking genioglossal EMG in sleep apnea patients versus normal controls (a neuromuscular compensatory mechanisms). J Clin Invest 1992;89:1571–9.

12. Horner RL. Motor control of the pharyngeal musculature and implications for the pathogenesis of obstructive sleep apnea. Sleep 1996;19(10):827–53.

13. Tangel DJ, Mezzanotte WS, White DP. The influence of NREM sleep on the activity of the palatoglossus and levator palatinin muscles in normal men. J Appl Physiol (1985) 1995;78:689–95.

14. Khoo M. Determinants of ventilatory instability and variability. Respir Physiol 2000;122:167–82.

15. Younes M, Ostrowski M, Thompson W, et al. Chemical control stability in patients with obstructive sleep apnea. Am J Respir Crit Care Med 2001;163(5):1181–90.

16. Sands SA, Mebrate Y, Edwards BA, et al. Resonance as the mechanism of daytime periodic breathing in patients with heart failure. Am J Respir Crit Care Med 2017;195(2):237–46.

17. Hudgel DW, Devadatta P, Quadri M, et al. Mechanism of sleep-induced periodic breathing in convalescing stroke patients and healthy elderly subjects. Chest 1993;104(5):1503–10.

18. Berry RB, Gleeson K. Respiratory arousal from sleep: mechanisms and significance. Sleep 1997;20(8):654–75.

19. Younes M. Role of arousals in the pathogenesis of obstructive sleep apnea. Am J Respir Crit Care Med 2004;169(5):623–33.

20. Edwards BA, Eckert DJ, McSharry DG, et al. Clinical predictors of the respiratory arousal threshold in patients with obstructive sleep apnea. Am J Respir Crit Care Med 2014;190(11):1293–300.

21. Gleeson K, Zwillich CW, WHite DP. The influence of increasing ventilatory effort on arousal from sleep. Am Rev Respir Dis 1990;142:295–300.

22. Stanchina M, Malhotra A, Fogel RB, et al. Genioglossus muscle responsiveness to chemical and mechanical loading during NREM sleep. Am J Respir Crit Care Med 2002;165:945–9.

23. Jordan AS, Wellman A, Heinzer RC, et al. Mechanisms used to restore ventilation after partial upper airway collapse during sleep in humans. Thorax 2007;62(10):861–7.

24. Edwards BA, Sands SA, Owens RL, et al. The combination of supplemental oxygen and a hypnotic markedly improves obstructive sleep apnea in patients with a mild to moderate upper airway collapsibility. Sleep 2016;39(11):1973–83.

25. Landry SA, Joosten SA, Sands SA, et al. Response to a combination of oxygen and a hypnotic as treatment for obstructive sleep apnoea is predicted by a patient's therapeutic CPAP requirement. Respirology 2017;22(6):1219–24.

26. Owens RL, Edwards BA, Sands SA, et al. The classical Starling resistor model often does not predict inspiratory airflow patterns in the human upper airway. J Appl Physiol (1985) 2014;116(8):1105–12.

27. Azarbarzin A, Sands SA, Marques M, et al. Palatal prolapse as a signature of expiratory flow limitation and inspiratory palatal collapse in patients with obstructive sleep apnoea. Eur Respir J 2018;51(2) [pii:1701419].

28. Weaver EM, Maynard C, Yueh B. Survival of veterans with sleep apnea: continuous positive airway pressure versus surgery. Otolaryngol Head Neck Surg 2004;130(6):659–65.

29. Kezirian EJ. Nonresponders to pharyngeal surgery for obstructive sleep apnea: insights from drug-induced sleep endoscopy. Laryngoscope 2011;121(6):1320–6.

30. Strollo PJ Jr, Malhotra A. Stimulating therapy for obstructive sleep apnoea. Thorax 2016;71(10):879–80.

31. Strollo PJ Jr, Soose RJ, Maurer JT, et al. Upper-airway stimulation for obstructive sleep apnea. N Engl J Med 2014;370(2):139–49.

32. Malhotra A. Hypoglossal-nerve stimulation for obstructive sleep apnea. N Engl J Med 2014;370(2):170–1.

33. Li Y, Ye J, Han D, et al. Physiology-based modeling may predict surgical treatment outcome for obstructive sleep apnea. J Clin Sleep Med 2017;13(9):1029–37.

34. Edwards BA, Connolly JG, Campana LM, et al. Acetazolamide attenuates the ventilatory response to arousal in patients with obstructive sleep apnea. Sleep 2013;36(2):281–5.

35. Eckert DJ, Owens RL, Kehlmann GB, et al. Eszopiclone increases the respiratory arousal threshold

and lowers the apnoea/hypopnoea index in obstructive sleep apnoea patients with a low arousal threshold. Clin Sci (Lond) 2011;120(12):505–14.

36. Smales ET, Edwards BA, Deyoung PN, et al. Trazodone effects on obstructive sleep apnea and non-REM arousal threshold. Ann Am Thorac Soc 2015; 12(5):758–64.

37. Wellman A, Edwards BA, Sands SA, et al. A simplified method for determining phenotypic traits in patients with obstructive sleep apnea. J Appl Physiol (1985) 2013;114(7):911–22.

38. Sands SA, Edwards BA, Terrill PI, et al. Phenotyping pharyngeal pathophysiology using polysomnography in patients with obstructive sleep apnea. Am J Respir Crit Care Med 2018;197(9):1187–97.

39. Terrill PI, Edwards BA, Nemati S, et al. Quantifying the ventilatory control contribution to sleep apnoea using polysomnography. Eur Respir J 2014;45(2): 408–18.

40. Orr JE, Sands SA, Edwards BA, et al. Measuring loop gain via home sleep testing in patients with obstructive sleep apnea. Am J Respir Crit Care Med 2018;197(10):1353–5.

41. Montesi SB, Bajwa EK, Malhotra A. Biomarkers of sleep apnea. Chest 2012;142(1):239–45.

42. Keenan BT, Kim J, Singh B, et al. Recognizable clinical subtypes of obstructive sleep apnea across international sleep centers: a cluster analysis. Sleep 2018;41(3).

43. Pien GW, Ye L, Keenan BT, et al. Changing faces of obstructive sleep apnea: treatment effects by cluster designation in the Icelandic sleep apnea cohort. Sleep 2018;41(3).

44. Zinchuk AV, Jeon S, Koo BB, et al. Polysomnographic phenotypes and their cardiovascular implications in obstructive sleep apnoea. Thorax 2018; 73(5):472–80.

45. Edwards BA, O'Driscoll DM, Ali A, et al. Aging and sleep: physiology and pathophysiology. Semin Respir Crit Care Med 2010;31(5):618–33.

46. Edwards BA, Wellman A, Sands SA, et al. Obstructive sleep apnea in older adults is a distinctly different physiological phenotype. Sleep 2014; 37(7):1227–36.

47. Kobayashi M, Namba K, Tsuiki S, et al. Clinical characteristics in two subgroups of obstructive sleep apnea syndrome in the elderly: comparison between cases with elderly and middle-age onset. Chest 2010;137(6):1310–5.

48. Punjabi NM, Caffo BS, Goodwin JL, et al. Sleep-disordered breathing and mortality: a prospective cohort study. PLoS Med 2009;6(8):e1000132.

49. Lavie P, Herer P, Peled R, et al. Mortality in sleep apnea patients: a multivariate analysis of risk factors [see comments]. Sleep 1995;18(3):149–57.

50. Stanchina M, Robinson K, Corrao W, et al. Clinical use of loop gain measures to determine continuous positive airway pressure efficacy in patients with complex sleep apnea. A pilot study. Ann Am Thorac Soc 2015;12(9):1351–7.

51. Pepin JD, Woehrle H, Liu D, et al. Adherence to positive airway therapy after switching from CPAP to ASV: a Big data analysis. J Clin Sleep Med 2018; 14(1):57–63.

52. Joosten SA, Leong P, Landry SA, et al. Loop gain predicts the response to upper airway surgery in patients with obstructive sleep apnea. Sleep 2017; 40(7).

53. Orr JE, Smales C, Alexander TH, et al. Treatment of OSA with CPAP is associated with improvement in PTSD symptoms among veterans. J Clin Sleep Med 2017;13(1):57–63.

54. Pillar G, Malhotra A, Lavie P. Post-traumatic stress disorder and sleep-what a nightmare! Sleep Med Rev 2000;4(2):183–200.

55. Malhotra A, Morrell MJ, Eastwood PR. Update in respiratory sleep disorders: epilogue to a modern review series. Respirology 2018;23(1):16–7.

56. Lebkuchen A, Carvalho VM, Venturini G, et al. Metabolomic and lipidomic profile in men with obstructive sleep apnoea: implications for diagnosis and biomarkers of cardiovascular risk. Sci Rep 2018; 8(1):11270.

57. Bhattacharjee R, Khalyfa A, Khalyfa AA, et al. Exosomal cargo properties, endothelial function and treatment of obesity hypoventilation syndrome: a proof of concept study. J Clin Sleep Med 2018;14(5): 797–807.

58. Xue J, Zhou D, Poulsen O, et al. Intermittent hypoxia and hypercapnia accelerate atherosclerosis partially via trimethylamine-oxide. Am J Respir Cell Mol Biol 2017;57(5):581–8.

59. Malhotra A, Crocker ME, Willes L, et al. Patient engagement using new technology to improve adherence to positive airway pressure therapy: retrospective analysis. Chest 2018;153(4):843–50.

60. Weaver TE, Grunstein RR. Adherence to continuous positive airway pressure therapy: the challenge to effective treatment. Proc Am Thorac Soc 2008;5(2): 173–8.

61. Hoy CJ, Venelle M, Douglas NJ. Can CPAP use be improved? Am J Respir Crit Care Med 1997;155: 304A.

62. Hoy CJ, Vennelle M, Kingshott RN, et al. Can intensive support improve continuous positive airway pressure use in patients with the sleep apnea/hypopnea syndrome? Am J Respir Crit Care Med 1999; 159(4 Pt 1):1096–100.

Precision Medicine for Sleep Loss and Fatigue Management

Luis E. Pichard, MHS, PhD[a],*, Guido Simonelli, MD[b], Lindsay Schwartz, PhD[c],
Thomas J. Balkin, PhD[b], Steven Hursh, PhD[c]

KEYWORDS

- Sleep - Insufficiency - Loss - Fatigue - Performance - Management - Modeling

KEY POINTS

- Sleep loss and/or sleep insufficiency has many causes, it is a widespread phenomenon, and has short- and long-term consequences.
- Consequences to sleep loss are not homogenous across populations and many individual traits have been linked to resiliency and/or susceptibility to sleep loss.
- There are no quantifiable biomarkers for sleep loss. As such, mitigations are aimed at restoring daytime function.
- Decrements in cognitive performance have led the way to objectively assess sleep sufficiency.
- Maintenance of cognitive performance, a day-to-day necessary function, is the primary outcome used in predictive models aimed at fatigue management caused by sleep insufficiency.

CAUSE OF SLEEP LOSS

Despite a growing body of scientific literature describing an ever-widening array of short-term behavioral deficits and long-term pathologies that are associated with sleep loss, and despite public health campaigns and the continuing efforts of such groups as the National Sleep Foundation, the American Academy of Sleep Medicine, and the National Institutes of Health, acute and chronic sleep loss remains an expanding widespread phenomenon.[1] Insufficient sleep is common, with approximately 25% of adults reporting sleep-related complaints at any given time.[2] The causes of insufficient sleep may result from a variety of factors, including medical conditions, sleep disorders, and occupation.[3] Sleep disorders, such as sleep disordered breathing, insomnia, and restless legs syndrome, can lead to insufficient sleep.[4] Medical conditions, such as musculoskeletal disorders including arthritis, fibromyalgia, or chronic back pain, can also disrupt sleep and lead to insufficient sleep.[5–7] The underlying mechanisms by which these disorders and medical conditions

Conflicts of Interest: S. Hursh is the inventor of the SAFTE model and SleepTank and the Institutes for Behavior Resources, Inc, sells products using the models.

Disclaimer: Material has been reviewed by the Walter Reed Army Institute of Research. There is no objection to its presentation and/or publication. The opinions or assertions contained herein are the private views of the authors, and are not to be construed as official, or as reflecting true views of the Department of the Army or the Department of Defense. The investigators have adhered to the policies for protection of human subjects as prescribed in AR 70–25.

[a] Division of Pulmonary and Critical Care Medicine, Department of Medicine, The Johns Hopkins University School of Medicine, 5501 Hopkins Bayview Circle, Baltimore, MD 21224, USA; [b] Behavioral Biology Branch, Walter Reed Army Institute of Research, 503 Robert Grant Avenue, Silver Spring, MD 20910, USA; [c] Institutes for Behavior Resources, Inc, 2104 Maryland Avenue, Baltimore, MD 21218, USA

* Corresponding author. Shush Performance Technologies, Inc., 626C Admiral Drive, #528, Annapolis, Maryland 21401, USA.

E-mail addresses: Luis.E.Pichard@gmail.com; Luis.Pichard@ShushPerformance.com

1556-407X/19/© 2019 Elsevier Inc. All rights reserved.

curtail sleep have been described elsewhere in this series. Lifestyle and occupational factors include shift work, long work hours, jet lag, and irregular schedules. Other lifestyle factors, such as sleep habits, timing of exercise, and diet, can also lead to insufficient sleep by diminishing sleep's restorative value (ie, worsening sleep quality). The underlying mechanisms by which lifestyle and occupational factors may lead to insufficient sleep include shortened sleep duration, increased sleep fragmentation, and circadian misalignment. Short sleep duration occurs when individuals reduce quantitatively or qualitatively their sleep opportunity. From a lifestyle/occupational standpoint, this is common in individuals with early shifts, long work hours, and long commutes. For instance, data on 6338 working adults from the National Health and Nutrition Examination Survey indicated that the prevalence of short sleep duration was twice as high in night shift workers.[8] Another study showed that those who worked an average of 55 hours per week or more are 2.5 times more likely to be short sleepers than those who work standard work weeks (35–40 hours).[9] In adults and adolescents it has also been shown that longer commutes are associated with shorter sleep.[10,11] A precision sleep medicine approach for sleep loss takes into consideration that consequences of sleep loss, sleep need, and efficacy of mitigation strategies to cope with insufficient sleep vary among individuals.

CONSEQUENCES OF SLEEP LOSS

Regardless of the underlying cause, accumulated chronic sleep loss is thought to have widespread and variegated consequences, including increased risk of atherosclerosis and cardiovascular disease[12,13]; increased rate of weight gain; and associated health risks, such as diabetes and cancer,[14] increased likelihood of Alzheimer disease,[15] impaired immune function,[16–21] and increased mortality[22,23] (to name but a few). Furthermore, individuals who obtain sufficient sleep have better cognitive functioning than those whose sleep is insufficient.[24] Findings from studies where the effects of sleep loss were assessed invariably show that it results in impaired performance on a wide variety of cognitive measures.[24] Additionally, because the spectrum of cognitive abilities impacted is broad, it is logical to hypothesize that one or more of the brain functions impacted by sleep loss are common to most types of cognitive performance (or are at least commonly reflected on tests of cognitive performance). For example, slowed response speed, difficulty concentrating, and reductions in vigilance and alertness[25,26]

underlie, or are a critical component of, performance on virtually all cognitive tasks. Functional neuroimaging studies have revealed that sleep loss results in relative deactivation of the brain, with heteromodal-associated areas, such as the prefrontal cortex (ie, those cortical regions that mediate the highest-order executive functions) especially impacted.[24,27] Consistent with these findings, sleep loss has been shown to degrade higher-order cognitive functions, such as creativity, divergent reasoning, and innovation, and planning, decision-making, and rule-based or convergent reasoning.[26,28] In general, measures of cognitive performance for which attention/vigilance are critical seem to be especially sensitive to sleep loss.[24]

INTERINDIVIDUAL RESPONSIVITY TO SLEEP LOSS

Healthy adults typically carry some level of "sleep debt"[29] that is paid down if they are afforded the opportunity and/or the proper motivation to do so. Paying down sleep debt ostensibly results in a nightly total sleep time that reflects the optimal homeostatic balance between the restorative properties of nighttime sleep and the daytime expenditure of sleep-produced resources (with, of course, sleep duration and timing also mediated by the circadian rhythm of alertness).[30] Even at equal levels of sleep debt, individuals respond differently to sleep loss, which may have implications for precision-based sleep medicine. In fact, there seems to be a normal distribution of neurobehavioral responsivity to lack of sleep.[31] Although there are considerable interindividual differences, the extent to which sleep loss impacts performance within individuals is fairly stable. Several studies have documented traitlike individual differences in terms of the magnitude of sleep need, the extent to which fatigue and sleepiness manifest, and neurobiologic vulnerability to lack of sleep.[32–36] That interindividual neurobiologic differences are not uniquely explained by sleep history suggests a genetic basis, a supposition that is supported by findings from several studies.[33,35,36] For example, Kuna and colleagues[37] showed that performance during sleep deprivation is highly heritable. When comparing monozygotic and dizygotic twins, monozygotic twins showed a significantly higher concordance following 38-hour sleep deprivation period, and concordance rates were similar to those expected for repeated intraindividual trials. Other studies have revealed several polymorphisms of clock genes that are determinants of interindividual variability in performance and recovery sleep.[38–40] Furthermore, polymorphisms that alter molecular pathways, such as the adenosine pathway, have been shown to determine interindividual response variability to caffeine intake and to modulate performance during sleep deprivation.[41]

Age is another important factor determining individual responsivity to sleep loss. Younger individuals are more susceptible to sleep loss. Profound differences in sleep architecture have been demonstrated in humans and animals across life spans. Several hypotheses have been proposed to explain the greater susceptibility to sleep loss of younger individuals.[42,43] These hypotheses have been described in Zitting and colleagues,[42] and are outside of the scope of this review.

Finally, personality traits have also been identified as potential determinants of vulnerability/resilience to sleep loss. For example, there is a small body of literature that shows differences between introverts and extroverts.[44,45] In this study, extroverts demonstrated increased vulnerability to the effects of sleep loss after social interaction.[45] However, the extent to which phenotypic variability is mediated by the aforementioned putative predictors is unknown.

ASSESSMENT TOOLS FOR SLEEP LOSS

Taking into consideration the existence of large interindividual differences described previously, an ideal assessment tool would include sleep duration obtained by each individual relative to the duration of nightly sleep needed by each individual. Because an accurate, quantifiable biomarker of sleep debt level is yet to be discovered, in this section we describe some of the existing tools to measure and monitor sleep sufficiency. The examples of assessment tools for sleep loss described in this section are listed in **Table 1**, and the impacted cognitive abilities following sleep loss.

Both sleepiness and fatigue are impacted by insufficient sleep. Sleepiness varies systematically as a function of the daily sleep/wake cycle, but it is also a physiologic state that is mediated by circadian, homeostatic, rhythmic, and behavioral factors.[19] The Multiple Sleep Latency Test and the Maintenance of Wakefulness Test are generally considered the gold standard measures of sleepiness. Self-reported sleepiness measures, such as the Stanford Sleepiness Scale or the Karolinska Sleepiness Scale, quantify extant subjective sleepiness state.[46,47] In contrast, the Epworth Sleepiness Scale is a validated measure of chronic sleepiness level (ie, traitlike sleepiness).[48] Fatigue, however, which is less clearly defined, has been described as "weariness" related to a lack of motivation, weakness, or depleted energy,[20] or, alternatively, a failure to initiate or sustain tasks requiring motivation.[21] The most common measure of fatigue, the Fatigue Severity Scale, has been validated for the assessment and quantification of fatigue in healthy and clinical populations,[47] as has the Fatigue Assessment Scale.[49,50] Additionally, work-related fatigue is assessed with such measures as the Occupational Fatigue Exhaustion/Recovery Scale, which measure chronic and acute fatigue, and fatigue recovery.[51]

Monitoring sleep sufficiency is critical for operational performance. It has been argued that carrying a mild level of sleep debt is not necessarily a liability. In this view, there are progressively diminishing returns for extending sleep, and on a normal day-to-day basis there is a point at which it becomes more beneficial to remain awake and productive than to obtain additional sleep.[52] However, two recent studies showed that although sleep extension does little to improve alertness or performance on the next day, its benefits do

Table 1
Summary of examples of tools to assess sleep loss and examples of cognitive impairments associated with sleep loss

	Self-Reported	Objective	Cognitive Impaired Ability
Tool	Karolinska Sleepiness Scale	PSG	Ability to recognize failed solutions
	Stanford Sleepiness Scale	MWT	Ability to generate novel solutions
	Fatigue Severity Scale	Actigraphy	Anticipating problems
	Epworth Sleepiness Scale	PVT	Planning and prioritizing
			Risk assessments
			Problem-solving
			Vigilance
			Attention to detail
			Ability to multitask
			Concentration/focus
			Emotional stability
			Motivation

Abbreviations: MWT, maintenance of wakefulness task; PSG, polysomnography; PVT, psychomotor vigilance task.

manifest under subsequent challenge of extended wakefulness.[53,54] Therefore, sleep extension clearly enhances resilience to decrements in alertness and performance resulting from sleep loss. As such, models based on sleep history may help with fatigue-related decision making. These models are based on self-reported sleep and/or actigraphic sleep measures, and can vary substantially in terms of complexity. One example of a model based on self-reported sleep history is a simple rule of thumb approach that aims to identify fitness for work, the Prior Sleep Wake Model.[55] The Prior Sleep Wake Model is comprised of three simple calculations: prior sleep in the last 24 and 48 hours, and length of the wakefulness period from awakening to end of work. An individual is unfit for work if any of the following criteria is met: less than 5 hours sleep in prior 24 hours; less than 12 hours sleep in prior 48 hours; current time awake exceeds amount of sleep in prior 48 hours. The US Army's sleep management software (2B-Alert), which is under development, is another tool that provides real-time feedback based on sleep history and also provides intervention recommendations (ie, caffeine usage) for maintaining alertness.[56] An interesting feature of this tool, which applies the Unified Model of Performance (UMP), is its capability to learn and predict at an individualized level. The software learns from the individual and is able to provide personalized feedback that fits that individual's need, independently of the source of the potential interindividual variability (eg, genetic, age, personality).[57] Another example of a fatigue management tool is SleepTank, a model in which wakefulness drains, and sleep refills, a sleep reservoir in much the same way that a gas tank is emptied and refilled on an automobile.[58] A final example that monitors sleep sufficiency is Fatigue Science's Readiband, which determines sleep/wake history from wrist actigraphy and inputs this information into the US Army's Sleep, Activity, Fatigue, and Task Effectiveness (SAFTE) model.[59] The model then produces a nonindividualized performance prediction (ie, based on group sleep/performance data) that equates to sleep sufficiency (ie, considers sleep history relative to an average 8-hour sleep need[60]).

MITIGATING STRATEGIES

The causes of insufficient sleep may be related to an untreated sleep disorder. In those cases, there are different precision sleep medicine approaches that have been described in this series. When the underlying cause of insufficient sleep relates to lifestyle and occupational factors, there are several mitigating strategies that can be used,

especially when the sleep loss responds to operational demands that have inherently inflexible schedules.[3] For example, using the tools described previously, at an individualized level, it is possible to recommend interventions to sustain neurobehavioral performance based on the current sleep reservoir.[56] These interventions could be aimed at (1) increasing sleep opportunities, (2) improving sleep quality, and (3) mitigating the consequences of sleep loss.

Quantitatively, nonpharmacologic interventions aimed at increasing restorative sleep quantity and quality include: scheduling sufficient recovery sleep following a long workday, prophylactic naps in the operational environment, and/or extending sleep with the goal of banking/storing sleep in anticipation of a long workday.[53] Nonpharmacologic interventions include interventions aimed at maximizing the recuperative value of the sleep period. These interventions lead to increased sleep efficiency and promote a less fragmented sleep. Nonpharmacologic interventions are a heterogeneous category that encompasses interventions related to lifestyle factors (diet and exercise), the sleep environment, and to sleep per se (eg, auditory stimulation during sleep[61]). For example, there is growing evidence that sleep quality is impacted by the timing of meals, and the type of food consumed during those meals.[6] When comparing a high-fat diet with a high carbohydrate diet, those with a high carbohydrate consumption had significantly less slow wave sleep, which is strongly associated with restorative processes, in the first sleep cycle.[63] Meal timing has long been identified as a zeitgeber, and may help synchronize the circadian rhythm of alertness.[64] Furthermore, there is some evidence that food choice may interact with the timing of the food intake.[65] Physical activity has also been linked to improved sleep quality[66]; it has been suggested that in the context of high cognitive demand, maintaining an exercise routine improves sleep quality.[66] Providing a comfortable sleep environment that mitigates environmental disruptors (light, noise, temperature, and air quality) improves sleep quality.[67] Finally, interventions that use auditory closed-loop stimulation to augment restorative sleep show some promise.[61] In terms of pharmacologic interventions, the next 2B-Alert version will include individualized recommendations for caffeine intake that are based on the individual's sensitivity to sleep loss and his/her responsivity to caffeine.[68] However, it should be noted that interventions aimed at mitigating the consequences of sleep loss are self-limiting and not sustainable. For example, a recent study suggests waning effectiveness of daytime caffeine administration over several consecutive days of sleep restriction.[69]

FUTURE DIRECTIONS: INDIVIDUALIZED SLEEP, FATIGUE MANAGEMENT, AND PREDICTIVE MODELING

An accruing sleep debt unquestionably leads to fatigue and detriments in neurobehavioral performance.[31,70] As previously suggested by Dawson and colleagues,[71] perhaps the most important question in fatigue management is an individual's sleep debt, which determines not only their fitness-for-duty but also dictates their ability to sustain performance throughout their work shift. Unfortunately, as described in this article and others,[56] individual susceptibilities to sleep loss, and thus fitness-for-duty, needs treatment plans to be individualized. Although they are informative and useful for such tasks as work/rest schedule making, population-based models are of limited utility for predicting (and thus managing) operational performance at the level of the individual.

Data models, some with their proprietary sleep predictors, that proactively address fatigue based on planned sleep opportunities have clear advantages in preventing incidents and are key for fatigue risk management systems (FRMS). These are widely used in air, ground, and rail transportation industries. Models include Boeing Alertness Model, InterDynamics fatigue evaluation model, System for Aircrew Fatigue Evaluation (SAFE), McCauley and colleagues[72] model, Pulsar's Fatigue evaluation model, and the SAFTE and UMP models,[73] but to name a few. However, individual susceptibilities and/or sleep needs are not accounted for in most of these models. At present, only the UMP model has been individualized via the 2B-Alert application.[57] The operational metric for predicting performance is the psychomotor vigilance test (PVT), and although the PVT has been validated and correlated with some aspects of operational performance,[73,74] it may not necessarily be appropriate for predicting all of operational performance. Yet, studies have shown that predictions based on PVT metrics do provide statistically significant predictions of railroad accident risk and accident cost in an operational environment.[75,76]

The recent, massive expansion of wearable technology is creating unprecedented possibilities in terms of the measurement, monitoring, and prediction of operational performance at the individual level. Currently the relevant technologies (eg, Optalert and LifeBand/SmartCap systems) function in a primarily reactive fashion. That is, they are designed to identify signs of extant fatigue,

but they do not predict future fatigue (eg, whether an individual operator's fatigue level will remain at an acceptable level for the remainder of his/her 8-hour shift). Obviously, this approach may be less than ideal because, for example, a pilot that is already flying the plane cannot stop flying because of excessive fatigue.

Individualized sleep assessments, sleep loss, and fatigue management remains a work in progress. An ideal FRMS would include individualized predictive modeling based on sleep opportunity, sleep history, and individual differences in sensitivity/resilience to sleep loss; and would accordingly provide individualized countermeasure recommendations. At present, no fully functioning individualized FRMS exists, but progress is being made rapidly. But the 2B-Alert app, which proactively predicts performance at the individual level based on sleep history and individual sensitivity/resilience to sleep loss, and makes recommendations regarding optimal dosing and timing of caffeine to sustain performance, constitutes a significant step forward in the right direction.

REFERENCES

1. Colten HR, Altevogt BM, editors. Sleep disorders and sleep deprivation: an unmet public health problem. The National Academies Collection: Reports funded by National Institutes of Health; 2006.
2. Morin CM, Benca RM. Insomnia nature, diagnosis, and treatment. Handb Clin Neurol 2011;99:723–46.
3. Akerstedt T. Shift work and disturbed sleep/wakefulness. Sleep Med Rev 1998;2:117–28.
4. Young T, Peppard PE, Gottlieb DJ. Epidemiology of obstructive sleep apnea: a population health perspective. Am J Respir Crit Care Med 2002;165:1217–39.
5. Diaz-Piedra C, Di Stasi LL, Baldwin CM, et al. Sleep disturbances of adult women suffering from fibromyalgia: a systematic review of observational studies. Sleep Med Rev 2015;21:86–99.
6. Kim JH, Park EC, Lee KS, et al. Association of sleep duration with rheumatoid arthritis in Korean adults: analysis of seven years of aggregated data from the Korea National Health and Nutrition Examination Survey (KNHANES). BMJ Open 2016;6:e011420.
7. Marin R, Cyhan T, Miklos W. Sleep disturbance in patients with chronic low back pain. Am J Phys Med Rehabil 2006;85:430–5.
8. Yong LC, Li J, Calvert GM. Sleep-related problems in the US working population: prevalence and association with shiftwork status. Occup Environ Med 2017;74:93–104.

9. Virtanen M, Ferrie JE, Gimeno D, et al. Long working hours and sleep disturbances: the Whitehall II prospective cohort study. Sleep 2009;32:737–45.

10. Petrov ME, Weng J, Reid KJ, et al. Commuting and sleep: results from the Hispanic community health study/study of Latinos Sueno ancillary study. Am J Prev Med 2018;54:e49–57.

11. Pereira EF, Moreno C, Louzada FM. Increased commuting to school time reduces sleep duration in adolescents. Chronobiol Int 2014;31:87–94.

12. Knutsson A, Boggild H. Shiftwork and cardiovascular disease: review of disease mechanisms. Rev Environ Health 2000;15:359–72.

13. Knutsson A, Hallquist J, Reuterwall C, et al. Shiftwork and myocardial infarction: a case-control study. Occup Environ Med 1999;56:46–50.

14. Cappuccio FP, D'Elia L, Strazzullo P, et al. Quantity and quality of sleep and incidence of type 2 diabetes: a systematic review and meta-analysis. Diabetes Care 2010;33:414–20.

15. Musiek ES, Xiong DD, Holtzman DM. Sleep, circadian rhythms, and the pathogenesis of Alzheimer disease. Exp Mol Med 2015;47:e148.

16. Spiegel K, Sheridan JF, Van Cauter E. Effect of sleep deprivation on response to immunization. JAMA 2002;288:1471–2.

17. Lange T, Dimitrov S, Bollinger T, et al. Sleep after vaccination boosts immunological memory. J Immunol 2011;187:283–90.

18. Lange T, Perras B, Fehm HL, et al. Sleep enhances the human antibody response to hepatitis A vaccination. Psychosom Med 2003;65:831–5.

19. Patel SR, Malhotra A, Gao X, et al. A prospective study of sleep duration and pneumonia risk in women. Sleep 2012;35:97–101.

20. Prather AA, Hall M, Fury JM, et al. Sleep and antibody response to hepatitis B vaccination. Sleep 2012;35:1063–9.

21. Cohen S, Doyle WJ, Alper CM, et al. Sleep habits and susceptibility to the common cold. Arch Intern Med 2009;169:62–7.

22. Cappuccio FP, Cooper D, D'Elia L, et al. Sleep duration predicts cardiovascular outcomes: a systematic review and meta-analysis of prospective studies. Eur Heart J 2011;32:1484–92.

23. Cappuccio FP, D'Elia L, Strazzullo P, et al. Sleep duration and all-cause mortality: a systematic review and meta-analysis of prospective studies. Sleep 2010;33:585–92.

24. Killgore WD. Effects of sleep deprivation on cognition. Prog Brain Res 2010;185:105–29.

25. Lim J, Dinges DF. Sleep deprivation and vigilant attention. Ann N Y Acad Sci 2008;1129:305–22.

26. Lim J, Dinges DF. A meta-analysis of the impact of short-term sleep deprivation on cognitive variables. Psychol Bull 2010;136:375–89.

27. Harrison Y, Horne JA, Rothwell A. Prefrontal neuropsychological effects of sleep deprivation in young adults: a model for healthy aging? Sleep 2000;23:1067–73.

28. Harrison Y, Horne JA. The impact of sleep deprivation on decision making: a review. J Exp Psychol Appl 2000;6:236–49.

29. Basner M, Fomberstein KM, Razavi FM, et al. American time use survey: sleep time and its relationship to waking activities. Sleep 2007;30:1085–95.

30. Schwartz JR, Roth T. Neurophysiology of sleep and wakefulness: basic science and clinical implications. Curr Neuropharmacol 2008;6:367–78.

31. Goel N, Rao H, Durmer JS, et al. Neurocognitive consequences of sleep deprivation. Semin Neurol 2009;29:320–39.

32. Van Dongen HP, Bender AM, Dinges DF. Systematic individual differences in sleep homeostatic and circadian rhythm contributions to neurobehavioral impairment during sleep deprivation. Accid Anal Prev 2012;45(Suppl):11–6.

33. Van Dongen HP, Baynard MD, Maislin G, et al. Systematic interindividual differences in neurobehavioral impairment from sleep loss: evidence of trait-like differential vulnerability. Sleep 2004;27:423–33.

34. Van Dongen HP, Maislin G, Dinges DF. Dealing with inter-individual differences in the temporal dynamics of fatigue and performance: importance and techniques. Aviat Space Environ Med 2004;75:A147–54.

35. Goel N, Banks S, Lin L, et al. Catechol-O-methyltransferase Val158Met polymorphism associates with individual differences in sleep physiologic responses to chronic sleep loss. PLoS One 2011;6:e29283.

36. Goel N, Banks S, Mignot E, et al. DQB1*0602 predicts interindividual differences in physiologic sleep, sleepiness, and fatigue. Neurology 2010;75:1509–19.

37. Kuna ST, Maislin G, Pack FM, et al. Heritability of performance deficit accumulation during acute sleep deprivation in twins. Sleep 2012;35:1223–33.

38. Viola AU, Archer SN, James LM, et al. PER3 polymorphism predicts sleep structure and waking performance. Curr Biol 2007;17:613–8.

39. Groeger JA, Viola AU, Lo JC, et al. Early morning executive functioning during sleep deprivation is compromised by a PERIOD3 polymorphism. Sleep 2008;31:1159–67.

40. Maire M, Reichert CF, Gabel V, et al. Time-on-task decrement in vigilance is modulated by inter-individual vulnerability to homeostatic sleep pressure manipulation. Front Behav Neurosci 2014;8:59.

1. Bodenmann S, Hohoff C, Freitag C, et al. Polymorphisms of ADORA2A modulate psychomotor vigilance and the effects of caffeine on neurobehavioural performance and sleep EEG after sleep deprivation. Br J Pharmacol 2012;165: 1904–13.

2. Zitting KM, Munch MY, Cain SW, et al. Young adults are more vulnerable to chronic sleep deficiency and recurrent circadian disruption than older adults. Sci Rep 2018;8:11052.

3. Bliese PD, Wesensten NJ, Balkin TJ. Age and individual variability in performance during sleep restriction. J Sleep Res 2006;15:376–85.

4. Killgore WD, Richards JM, Killgore DB, et al. The trait of introversion-extraversion predicts vulnerability to sleep deprivation. J Sleep Res 2007;16: 354–63.

5. Rupp TL, Killgore WD, Balkin TJ. Socializing by day may affect performance by night: vulnerability to sleep deprivation is differentially mediated by social exposure in extraverts vs introverts. Sleep 2010;33: 1475–85.

6. Kaida K, Takahashi M, Akerstedt T, et al. Validation of the Karolinska sleepiness scale against performance and EEG variables. Clin Neurophysiol 2006; 117:1574–81.

7. MacLean AW, Fekken GC, Saskin P, et al. Psychometric evaluation of the Stanford sleepiness scale. J Sleep Res 1992;1:35–9.

8. Lapin BR, Bena JF, Walia HK, et al. The Epworth sleepiness scale: validation of one-dimensional factor structure in a large clinical sample. J Clin Sleep Med 2018;14:1293–301.

9. De Vries J, Michelson H, Van Heck GL, et al. Measuring fatigue in sarcoidosis: the fatigue assessment scale (FAS). Br J Health Psychol 2004;9: 279–91.

50. Michelson HJ, De Vries J, Van Heck GL. Psychometric qualities of a brief self-rated fatigue measure: the fatigue assessment scale. J Psychosom Res 2003; 54:345–52.

51. Winwood PC, Winefield AH, Dawson D, et al. Development and validation of a scale to measure work-related fatigue and recovery: the occupational fatigue exhaustion/recovery scale (OFER). J Occup Environ Med 2005;47:594–606.

52. Horne J. The end of sleep: 'sleep debt' versus biological adaptation of human sleep to waking needs. Biol Psychol 2011;87:1–14.

53. Rupp TL, Wesensten NJ, Bliese PD, et al. Banking sleep: realization of benefits during subsequent sleep restriction and recovery. Sleep 2009;32: 311–21.

54. Arnal PJ, Sauvet F, Leger D, et al. Benefits of sleep extension on sustained attention and sleep pressure before and during total sleep deprivation and recovery. Sleep 2015;38:1935–43.

55. Darwent D, Dawson D, Paterson JL, et al. Managing fatigue: it really is about sleep. Accid Anal Prev 2015;82:20–6.

56. Capaldi VF, Balkin TJ, Mysliwiec V. Optimizing sleep in the military: challenges and opportunities. Chest 2019;155:215–26.

57. Reifman J, Ramakrishnan S, Liu J, et al. 2B-alert app: a mobile application for real-time individualized prediction of alertness. J Sleep Res 2018;28(2): e12725.

58. Dorrian J, Hursh S, Waggoner L, et al. How much is left in your "sleep tank"? Proof of concept for a simple model for sleep history feedback. Accid Anal Prev 2019;126:177–83.

59. Mallis MM, Mejdal S, Nguyen TT, et al. Summary of the key features of seven biomathematical models of human fatigue and performance. Aviat Space Environ Med 2004;75:A4–14.

60. Hursh SR, Balkin TJ, Van Dongen HPA. Sleep and performance modeling. In: Kryger M, Roth T, Dement WC, editors. Principles and practice of sleep medicine. Philadelphia: Elsevier; 2017. p. 689–96.

61. Ngo HV, Miedema A, Faude I, et al. Driving sleep slow oscillations by auditory closed-loop stimulation-a self-limiting process. J Neurosci 2015;35:6630–8.

62. St-Onge MP, Mikic A, Pietrolungo CE. Effects of diet on sleep quality. Adv Nutr 2016;7:938–49.

63. Yajima K, Seya T, Iwayama K, et al. Effects of nutrient composition of dinner on sleep architecture and energy metabolism during sleep. J Nutr Sci Vitaminol (Tokyo) 2014;60:114–21.

64. Asher G, Sassone-Corsi P. Time for food: the intimate interplay between nutrition, metabolism, and the circadian clock. Cell 2015;161:84–92.

65. Afaghi A, O'Connor H, Chow CM. High-glycemic-index carbohydrate meals shorten sleep onset. Am J Clin Nutr 2007;85:426–30.

66. Wunsch K, Kasten N, Fuchs R. The effect of physical activity on sleep quality, well-being, and affect in academic stress periods. Nat Sci Sleep 2017;9: 117–26.

67. Caddick ZA, Gregory K, Arsintescu L, et al. A review of the environmental parameters necessary for an optimal sleep environment. Build Environ 2018;132: 11–20.

68. Reifman J, Kumar K, Wesensten NJ, et al. 2B-Alert web: an open-access tool for predicting the effects of sleep/wake schedules and caffeine consumption on neurobehavioral performance. Sleep 2016;39: 2157–9.

69. Doty TJ, So CJ, Bergman EM, et al. Limited efficacy of caffeine and recovery costs during and following 5 days of chronic sleep restriction. Sleep 2017;40.

70. Dinges DF, Pack F, Williams K, et al. Cumulative sleepiness, mood disturbance, and psychomotor

vigilance performance decrements during a week of sleep restricted to 4-5 hours per night. Sleep 1997; 20:267–77.

71. Dawson, McCulloch K. Managing fatigue: It's about sleep. Sleep Medicine Reviews 2005;9(5): 365–80.

72. McCauley P, Kalachev LV, Mollicone DJ, et al. Dynamic circadian modulation in a biomathematical model for the effects of sleep and sleep loss on waking neurobehavioral performance. Sleep 2013; 36:1987–97.

73. Lieberman HR, Bathalon GP, Falco CM, et al. The fog of war: decrements in cognitive performance and mood associated with combat-like stress. Aviat Space Environ Med 2005;76 C7–14.

74. Caldwell JA. Fatigue in aviation. Travel Med Infec Dis 2005;3:85–96.

75. Hursh SR, Raslear TG, Kaye AS, et a Validation and calibration of a fatigue assessmer tool for railroad work schedules, final repor Washington, DC: U.S. Department of Transporta tion; 2008.

76. Hursh SR, Fanzone JF, Raslear TG. Analysis of th relationship between operator effectiveness mea sures and economic impacts of rail accidents Washington, DC: U.S. Department of Transportatior 2011.

Moving?

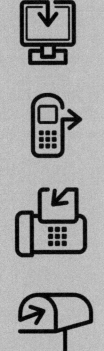